Dancing on Drugs

Dancing on Drugs
Risk, Health and Hedonism
in the British Club Scene

Fiona Measham, Judith Aldridge
and Howard Parker

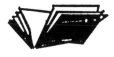

FREE ASSOCIATION BOOKS / LONDON / NEW YORK

First published in Great Britain 2001 by
FREE ASSOCIATION BOOKS
57 Warren Street
London W1T 5NR

Copyright © Fiona Measham, Judith Aldridge and Howard Parker 2001

ISBN 1 85343 512 0 pbk

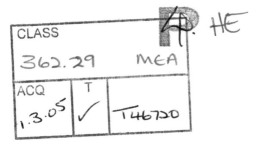

Designed, typeset and produced for
Free Association Books Ltd by Chase Publishing Services
Printed in the European Union by Antony Rowe Ltd, Chippenham, England

Contents

List of Tables

Acknowledgements

We must first thank the members of the fieldwork team. Their dedication and hard work involved a considerable sacrifice, as they worked diligently, smilingly, and reliably until the early hours of the morning, and with great skill and professionalism. We were privileged to have worked with such a team: Lucy Attenborough, Jon Breeze, Tony Bullock, Dean Herd, Tina James, Debbie Oates, Jaki Pugh, Craig Ruckledge and Chendi Ukwuoma.

We would like to express our gratitude to Dianne Moss, SPARC administrative secretary at the University of Manchester, who helped throughout the course of the fieldwork and also assisted in the preparation of the manuscript for this book. We were ably helped with the complicated task of collating and coding the vast amount of data collected by Nicola Elson and Rob Ralphs. We are grateful to the team at Medeval in Manchester who carried out the medical assessments, and in particular to Simon Cooper who liaised. Urine samples were analysed by Tony Tetlow and George Waite and the team at Hope Hospital in Salford. Our thanks to them for their enthusiasm towards our samples and their willingness to discuss urine in so much depth! We would like to thank the ESRC for funding the research.

Other people who assisted, advised or supported, or without whom this would have been a very different book include: Alex Aldridge, Bart Alexander, Dawn Cowdell, Forrest Frankovitch, Jane Hart, Marcus Hathaway, Rob McCracken, Maria Measham, Eddie Scouller, Colin Wilson, Janet Wolstenholme and the Quest regulars.

We would like to thank all the staff and management at the three fieldwork clubs who gave us access to their venues and gave of their work time in facilitating our research. We would particularly like to thank all the clubbers who participated in the various aspects of this study and without whom there would have been no study. They gave so willingly of their leisure time as respondents but also were enthusiastic about the importance of conducting studies such as this on dance drugs and dance clubs. We are appreciative of how forthcoming they were about their personal lives and amazed at how obliging they were in relation to the many different social and medical aspects of this study.

Finally, this is far from purely an academic study for the authors. Fiona Measham has been clubbing since the age of 13, working in clubs since the age of 15, and can still be spotted dancing in the odd club around town. This book is, therefore, dedicated to all clubbers, to everyone who has felt that moment when music, dancing, atmosphere and experience have melted into a moment of pure pleasure.

1 Excessive Appetites?[1] Young Britons and Recreational Drug Use

The UK now hosts the most drug-experienced youth and young adult population in Europe with only international neighbour Ireland even in the same league (ESPAD, 1997). Young Britons, using national samples, now take as many drugs as their peers in the USA (NHSDA, 1999; Ramsay and Partridge, 1999). Whilst there is a worrying deterioration in drug use orbiting around heroin and (crack) cocaine, the engine for this rise to the top of the illegal drug-use tables is *recreational* consumption involving cannabis, amphetamines, ecstasy and, increasingly, cocaine. This status of having the most drug-involved population may have been generated over the past 20 years but only became transparent during the 1990s as international comparisons became possible across the European Union (EMCDDA, 1999; Griffiths et al., 1997) and via the increasing harmonisation of drug indicators between the UK and USA.

This study explores the most serious end of the UK's recreational drug-using population. We focus on the minority who move beyond cannabis and include amphetamines, poppers, cocaine and especially ecstasy in their repertoires – the dance drug users.

In this chapter we begin by very briefly summarising the nature of adolescent drug trying and use in the UK. There is a substantive literature on under-sixteens and, to a lesser extent, under-eighteens. However because the focus of our study, the clubbers as dance drug users, are primarily in their late teens and twenties we attempt to describe the rates of drug use amongst this age group population in this chapter, exploring the cultural context for dance drug use in the next chapter. We can make only the broadest of summaries because once young people leave school at 16 and 18 young Britons scatter into an array of educational, training and employment or indeed unemployment situations making them extremely hard to recapture and research, certainly if we are looking for large representative samples. What does become apparent however is that whilst young adults are generally becoming more drug experienced, as an age group, they do not look like the profiles of clubbers generated so far. Clubbers are even more likely to be smokers, regular drinkers, cannabis users, triers of most drugs and users of the stimulant dance drug repertoire. We demonstrate this by reviewing current knowledge, based on a clutch of 1990s studies of customers of the night club–dance club scene.

Our final task in this chapter is to attempt to explain these differences between adolescent and young adult recreational drug users and the clubbers. Although the UK has a very drug-experienced adolescent population of 16- to 17-year-olds their overall drugs profiles are still benign or slight compared with the clubbers just a few years their senior. There are processes at work both in adolescence and during the post-adolescent transition period which explain how the clubbers became so drugs experienced so quickly. Much of this is about self-selection and being part of the much broader 'going out' sector amongst 17- to 30-year-olds. However we will suggest that many of the defining characteristics and drugs pathways the clubbers take are identifiable in earlier adolescence and become even more distinctive if and as they become regular clubbers.

Adolescent drug use across the 1990s

In due course the 1990s may well be seen as the decade when recreational drug use first became normalised. Normalisation is a process perspective, a relative concept. The changes in social attitudes and behaviour vis-à-vis, in this case, illegal drugs is controlled by the relevant population – today's youth and to some extent their elders. Smoking illustrates how dynamic normalisation is. Thus the less age-specific normalisation of tobacco use which occurred right across the last century is now being challenged by changing knowledge about health risks, the attitudes and behaviour of non-smokers, ex-smokers and often those who want to give up. Consequently smoking is becoming less socially acceptable in the wider population. Normalisation can be reversed therefore and so the day may thus come when a particular era of British youth rejects psycho-active drug use, thereby pushing back the normalisation process and redefining such drug taking as unacceptable and requiring effective sanction. If and when this occurs those who wish to continue using drugs will need to retreat into covert settings and become more socially organised to maintain their behaviour. They in turn become located in more subterranean or subcultural worlds – as indeed heroin or crack cocaine users are today – because their drug use and lifestyles are rejected, even abhorred, by many 'conventional' people including their peers.

The normalisation of recreational drug use gradually bedded-in right across the 1990s. We saw quite massive increases in the availability of street drugs and their accessibility to ordinary conventional youth. Similarly by whatever measure used, drug trying increased substantially. This is plotted in household surveys, school-based surveys and longitudinal studies. Even the official government household measure has monitored drug trying from being a minority to a majority activity. For instance, 16- to 24-year-olds in the past three bi-annual surveys have shown increases from 45 per cent (1994) to 48 per cent (1996) to

52 per cent reporting illicit drugs experience with the figure for young men now at 58 per cent (Ramsay and Partridge, 1999). The other key household survey for England using a larger sample in respect of the 11–35 age groups recorded lifetime rates of 58 per cent for 20- to 24-year-olds (64 per cent for males) in 1996. On 'recent use' the household surveys find one in five past-month users and one in four past-three month users in the 16–24 age group (HEA, 1999).

Sensitive, confidential school-based surveys administered directly by researchers find these high rates even amongst under-16-year-olds although these have largely taken place in Scotland and Northern England where rates are somewhat higher (e.g. Aldridge et al., 1999; Parker et al., 1998; Barnard et al., 1996; Meikle et al., 1996). More recent use for these mid-adolescents rises with age to around one in five regular recreational users by the late teens.

It may well be that lifetime trying rates will plateau at around six to seven in ten as the point is reached where the remainder of young Britons have absolutely no wish to take drugs in the same way they wish to avoid tobacco or meat. Indeed just as there are signs that in the United States today's adolescents are slightly less drug experienced than the previous age cohort now in their twenties (NHSDA, 1999; Office of National Drug Control Policy, 1999), so we are probably seeing the beginnings of a plateau or even down-turn in drug experimentation in the UK. Recent time series self-report surveys across England (Balding, 1999) and the UK (Plant and Miller, 2000) are showing falls in the drug experimentation of today's mid-adolescents compared with those of the early and mid-1990s.

This said, these studies offer only very basic measures of drug trying rather than more regular drug use which researchers have anyway struggled to measure effectively (Egginton et al., 2001; Aldridge et al., 1999). If for instance rates of regular use, dominated by cannabis, remain at around 20–25 per cent of the adolescent and twentysomething population, then again the normalisation process will go little further. One of the key theoretical questions underpinning this study is: what do the dance drug users mean for normalisation and, even more importantly, what impact will the drugwise (Parker et al., 1998), drug-experienced adolescents of the 1990s have on these processes as they cross into adulthood with all the traditional assumptions that they will 'settle down' and leave deviant behaviour behind them? If in fact many, because of normalisation, do not regard continuing drug use as problematic or unacceptable, then the recent and regular drug-use figures firstly for 19- to 24-year-olds and then 25- to 30-year-olds will rise. If this is dominated by cannabis then this drug is clearly being defined as different and free-standing by the drug-experienced population and 'tolerant' non-users. If other drugs become widely used and 'accepted' the debate about normalisation will need revisiting.

In summary, although the term normalisation seems to generate emotive responses in some commentators, it is the most parsimonious conceptualisation because if applied properly it covers availability, trying, rates of use, user population characteristics and cultural accommodation measures. Moreover it is a multi-dimensional, dynamic concept and so can be used to assess rejection and reduction as well as accommodation and increases in recreational drug taking.

Whether we utilise the term or not the UK has now become one of the most drug-experienced post-industrial societies. Across the 1990s street drugs have become widely available, trying rates have doubled, regular use rates increased and a plethora of qualitative studies and some surveys have noted the normative characteristics of the user population and the accommodation of 'sensible' recreational drug use by most (but not all) young Britons including many who do not take drugs themselves (Pirie and Worcester, 1999).

'Time out' consumers and venues

Although, in due course, this study will focus on the core elements of the dance club scene, there is no prospect of understanding clubbing and dance drug use without first situating the clubbers in the wider leisure–consumption–going out landscape. Essentially dance clubs and night clubs are part of a broader leisure industry which not only hosts illegal drug use but provides the key features for the ideal night out. 'Time out' is about meeting with friends and going out to 'town' – drinking, socialising, listening to music, dancing, meeting new people and partners – and only perhaps taking illegal drugs.

The British night club–dance club scene is not easy to describe briefly (see Chapter 2) because not only is it constructed on robust historical and cultural habits but it is, in post-modern times, evolving, diversifying and relocating continuously within a fast-moving industry. Distinctions between pubs and bars, night clubs and dance clubs, 'raves' and festivals are all blurring, even disintegrating and reformulating. The basic trend is to include more and more elements of the 'ideal' time out episode in one venue or, more often, small dedicated area. This is increasingly a commercially-led evolution and market knowledge designs the ideal mix of entertainment–dancing–alcohol–food–sex and, more covertly, drugs.

Thus although the UK's official 4,000 night clubs attract 16 million club visits a year and according to leisure forecasters Mintel one in two 18- to 24-year-olds are regular clubbers (Finch, 1999), this categorisation falls far short of including the range of leisure locations where young people may use drugs as part of their 'time out'. Dancing on drugs for instance occurs at dance events which use metamorphosed leisure centres or empty warehouses, in café bars with alcohol licensing extensions, at festivals and pay parties, private parties, celebrations and so on.

Although, as we shall see in the next chapter, there are groups of ecstasy users who celebrate the absence of alcohol from their venues, we cannot adequately understand clubbing without continuous reference to alcohol (Measham et al.,

1998a). Its sale and consumption underpins the commercial success of most 'public' bars, café bars and clubs which are, for millions of young Britons, the venues where they congregate for their 'time out'.

In short, any social scientific analysis of clubbers and dance drug users must be located in the lifestyles of today's youth and the 'time out' leisure venues they frequent. One aspect of the normalisation of recreational drug use is how it co-habits with smoking tobacco and drinking alcohol. This process may be more 'advanced' in the UK than elsewhere and for reasons we do not fully understand, but it is being widely recognised as a global phenomenon in post-industrial societies. A study of nightlife in nine European cities (Athens (Greece), Berlin (Germany), Coimbra (Portugal), Modena (Italy), Nice (France), Manchester (UK), Palma (Spain), Utrecht (Netherlands) and Vienna (Austria)) found a great deal of symmetry. Over 2,500 participating young adults and twenty- and thirtysomethings (mean 21.8 years), questioned in a variety of ways in each city, largely concurred that the key reasons for going out were, in order of priority (but all important): to meet friends, to listen to music, to escape daily routine, to dance, to look for a partner, to look for sex and to take drugs. Yet all this must be framed with alcohol. Alcohol drives the bar and club culture which underpins these nights out, allowing circuit drinking and thus movement between nearby venues. Alcohol was nominated as far and away the samples' favourite drug followed by cannabis, ecstasy, cocaine and tobacco (Calafat, 1998).

Finally this study also reminds us of the way youth transitions are changing for young Europeans with the journey from adolescence to full adult citizenship being longer and more uncertain (Miles, 2000). Marriage and parenting are increasingly delayed and career 'choices' more fluid. The financial pressure to remain living at home well into the twenties is strong. This in itself may make 'time out' functional for middle-aged parents and energetic twentysomethings alike!

Psycho-active drug use amongst young adults

It is important for our analysis to assess the extent to which the clubbers–dance drug users are part of or apart from the social attitudes and habits of the larger post-adolescent and young adult population. Do we see their drug profiles as an extension of endemic recreational drug use in the wider population or as outside the norm and normative and thus inviting the use of deviancy perspectives and subcultural theories? Subcultural perspectives dominated explanations of previous post-war youth formations, although some commentators now see such perspectives as obsolete in post-modern times (Furlong and Cartmel, 1997).

Traditionally the criminological and life transitions literature has emphasised the importance of 'settling down' in the early twenties. Apart from a minority of 'career' deviants, delinquency and drug misuse (Graham and Bowling, 1995) fall away as young adults either mature out or become constrained by the responsibilities of work, family, parenting and so on. There is still possible evidence of this. In the mid-1990s the Scottish Crime Survey (a household survey) found 37 per cent of young men and 21 per cent of women of between 20 and 24 years had had an illicit drug in the past year but the rate more than halved for 25- to 29-year-olds (Scottish Office, 1997).

In this section we look briefly at the limited research data on the drugs habits of the clubbers' peers – the twentysomethings. The evidence is, as we shall see, equivocal. On the one hand at a population level drug use rates are far *lower* than those found amongst the clubbers but on the other hand there are clear signs that young adults are becoming more drug experienced than their predecessors and again as part of a wider pattern of psycho-active consumption including alcohol.

The most substantive cluster of research studies around the most obviously easy to capture group – university students – has been conducted by self-report, confidential or anonymous surveys. There has been a national survey (Webb et al., 1996) of 3,075 second-year undergraduates (mean age 20.9 years) and time series surveys of medical students (Ashton and Kamali, 1995; Birch et al., 1999).

Overall the key findings were that university students include a significant minority of heavy drinkers, a majority of regular drinkers and around 60 per cent have tried illicit drugs, primarily cannabis of whom 20 per cent of the sample were regular users. For incoming medical students the rates of drug use have more than doubled since the mid-1980s. All these studies make the point that the heavy drinkers–drug users tend to be 'risk takers', as measured on recognised psychological scales, who in the main began these drinking–drug taking careers during adolescence but whilst showing signs of everyday anxiety and stress. This did not relate to their alcohol or drug use which was defined as hedonistic.

Only a minority of dance drug triers were found in the national survey, around 13–18 per cent (lifetime rates LSD 18 per cent, ecstasy 13 per cent, poppers 15 per cent) but with only around 3 per cent being regular (at least once a week) users and around 6 per cent, at most, occasional users (Webb et al., 1996).

A smaller survey of university students (n=348) found that 96 per cent had drunk alcohol in the past 12 months and that of this group 22 per cent drank at least once a day and 62 per cent more than once a week. Just over half smoked tobacco. This study found slightly higher rates of drug taking than the other student surveys with around 10 per cent (over 12 per cent for males) being dance drug users. The authors' normalisation thesis was tested by looking for differential characteristics between psycho-active drug users and abstainers including health, personality and psychotic measures. They found no significant differences and concluded that normalisation was complete in respect of illicit drug use which has 'become part of the lifestyle of a significant and non-deviant proportion of students' (Makhoul et al., 1998).

An interview-based survey of 905 students from ten UK universities during 1999 produced similar results. This sample was characterised by a commitment to personal and career success which they felt higher education offered. Despite the financial pressures of funding their college life, over two-thirds spent more than £10 a week on alcohol and the norm for entertainment primarily for 'going out' was between £10 and £15 per week.

The lifetime drugs rates in this study were lower than for the other studies at around 40 per cent. This varied greatly between universities with small campus universities having lower rates and the urban 'city' universities having far higher rates of over 60 per cent. It may well be that this is partly a process of self-selection, with those who value the going out–time out lifestyle opting for metropolitan sites and those enjoying a quieter life preferring green fields or small town colleges.

However although rates of drug-taking experience were lower in this study another dimension of normalisation was evident. The normalisation of 'sensible' recreational drug use requires the non-drug users and users to co-exist socially. If the users are rejected we do not have an important plank of normalisation in place (Parker et al., 1998). This student sample was quite clear however that this inter-tolerance defined their population. They voiced a strong commitment to tolerance of other people's lifestyles, particularly in respect of sexuality and drug use. Over half (52 per cent) had friends who used drugs *regularly*. This was seen as unproblematic because of the sample's high degree of tolerance. The only thing they did not tolerate was intolerance itself (Pirie and Worcester, 1999).

Because young adults are 'scattered' they are difficult to investigate. In the absence of infinite research resources the most effective monitoring tool we have is the household survey. Although such surveys produce some under-reporting and are ineffective for finding problematic drug users, say of heroin or crack cocaine, household surveys are particularly cost-effective at finding recreational drug use in the wider population. The British Crime Surveys of the 1990s have all documented the steady growth in drug trying across the last decade. For England and Wales using a sample of around 2,500 16- to 29-year-olds we can see (Table 1.1) how lifetime use has been growing right across the key age range. The same general trend is evident using the 'past month' measure. Importantly the BCS confirms that those who go out regularly, drinking, have far higher rates of drug use and that this population comes from all socio-economic groups, particularly the affluent middle-class sector. Almost by definition because they are out so often, dance drug users will be under-repre-sented in such surveys.

The other large household survey undertaken via government found rather higher rates – and even in the mid-1990s. The Health Education Authority's (1999) survey in 1996 involved numerous sensitive drugs questions. It found that 54 per cent of 16- to 19-year-olds, 58 per cent of 19- to 24-year-olds and 52 per cent of 25- to 29-year-olds had ever tried drugs but with no less than 39 per cent of 16- to 19-year-olds, 33 per cent of 20- to 24-year-olds and 23 per cent of 25- to 29-year-olds having had a drug in the past year. Past month drug use was at 21 per cent for 16- to 24-year-olds but only 12 per cent for 25- to 29-year-olds. On the one hand this could reflect the 'settling down' process in the mid-twenties and on the other it may be the frontier between a generation who grew up without the ready availability and social use of drugs and those who did – the children of the Nineties.

Table 1.1   **Summary of British Crime Survey drugs prevalence rates**

Ages	Lifetime Prevalence (%)			Past Month Use (%)		
	1994	1996	1998	1994	1996	1998
16–19	46	45	49	20	19	22
20–24	44	49	55	15	18	17
25–29	39	41	45	9	10	11

(Adapted from British Crime Survey 1999)

Focusing on the dance drugs in these general population studies, we find that whilst well over 80 per cent in the HEA study said it would be easy to get amphetamines and ecstasy, the rates of actual consumption for 10- to 24-year-olds was around 16 per cent (24 per cent in BCS) for amphetamines and 7 per cent for ecstasy (12 per cent in BCS). Cocaine had been tried by 9 per cent of this age group in the 1998 BCS. Rates of recent use were a few per cent lower.

Finally, whilst gender differences are minimal in adolescent drug-using populations, we find gendered drug use emerging in young adulthood with higher rates of drug experimentation and use amongst adult males than females. In the BCS (Ramsay and Partridge, 1999) 64 per cent of males in their early twenties had ever taken a drug, 37 per cent in the past year and 25 per cent in the past month, all several per cent higher than for women.

In summary there are clear signs of an increase in recreational drug use amongst post-adolescents and twentysomethings at the beginning of the new millennium. The regular use of cannabis is far more prevalent than dance drug use however. Whilst somewhere around 20–25 per cent of this age group, particularly males, use cannabis, 'time out' dance drug use seems to involve under 10 per cent in the populations sampled. Importantly their most used psychoactive drug continues to be alcohol.

Upon this backcloth we can now look specifically at the drug-taking profiles of 1990s clubbers.

Drugs profiles of clubbers

In the UK

Whilst we are a long way from being able to generalise accurately about the drug-taking profiles of clubbers, several studies indicate that they are far more drug experienced than the general young adult population in the UK.

Forsyth (1998) interviewed 135 'ravers' who attended dance clubs in the West End of Glasgow. They had a mean age of 24 years and 70 per cent of the sample were twentysomethings. Over 80 per cent were single (only 14 had children) and were 'in a transitory life stage, usually between parental home and their own permanent home or between school and lifetime occupation'. Whilst 40 per cent were officially unemployed, over a quarter were in full-time education. Most were frequent users of alcohol, tobacco and the 'ubiquitous' cannabis. They were also highly drug experienced with lifetime 'ever tried' illicit drug-taking rates over 90 per cent for cannabis, amphetamines, LSD and ecstasy and with similar rates for past year use. Over 70 per cent had tried cocaine with a past year rate of 59 per cent. Moreover this sample could be described as poly drug users in that they used numerous different drugs on different occasions but often combined them on a night out (Hammersley et al., 1999).

A study by Akram (1997) in Nottingham produced remarkably similar results based on interviews with 125 dance drug users. Again we find extremely high lifetime prevalence rates for the dance drugs (amphetamines 98 per cent, ecstasy 96 per cent, LSD 91 per cent, cocaine 81 per cent).

A survey by Release (1997) of 496 dance event attendees in different parts of the country again found the 15–30 age profile, a wide variety of socio-economic backgrounds and the strong presence of people in further and higher education. Again lifetime drug-trying rates were exceptionally high with cannabis, ecstasy, amphetamines and LSD all over 80 per cent and cocaine at 62 per cent. Of particular importance was that these rates were as high for the 15- to 19-year-old (n = 153) sub sample as their elders. These respondents also had a pick 'n' mix approach to drug use, combining alcohol and tobacco with other drugs and using different drugs or combinations in different settings. So whilst most nominated cannabis as their favourite drug generally, ecstasy was their specific favourite to go out dancing on.

A qualitative study in Northern Ireland (Belfast) based on confidential in-depth interviews with 98 ecstasy users (mean age 25 years) again found very sophisticated drugs careers and regular stimulant use amongst the sample. Although not interviewed in club venues this group were experienced clubbers. They began using ecstasy at around 21 and most had used it for at least four years. There was no clear regularity of use pattern and indeed diversity defined the overall picture. All the sample had taken cannabis and a third were current daily users. With 44 per cent having taken cocaine, 93 per cent amphetamines, 97 per cent LSD and 88 per cent nitrite poppers, we again find a picture of 'serious' recreational drug use with the mixing of alchol and ecstasy widespread and poly drug use common.

Although there was a minority of 'delinquent' males in this sample for whom clubbing or 'raving' was part of their broader lifestyle, most were in work (57 per cent) and half were described as 'middle class' (McElrath and McEvoy, 1999).

In 1996 over 4,000 readers responded to a *Mixmag* survey providing details of their dance drug use: 97 per cent were regular clubbers, 81 per cent of whom were current ecstasy users with two-thirds of the sample reporting they took ecstasy at least once a fortnight. Moreover over 40 per cent of the sample said they had first taken ecstasy more than four years ago and 31 per cent said they planned to continue usage for at least another four years (Petridis, 1996). A further survey, via distribution of the magazine in 1999, received over a thousand responses. Clearly, using a self-selecting sample, the authors emphasised the risks and costs of dance drug use evident from their results (Winstock, 2000). Their respondents reported regular poly drug use, bingeing on ecstasy, using stimulant drugs as a weight reduction measure and using tranquillisers as a 'come down' drug. Again this sample were very 'lifetime' drug experienced.

With regional surveys in Wales (Handy et al., 1998) and Manchester (Sherlock in Calafat, 1998) producing similar profiles, a consistent picture builds up: young adult clubbers have florid drug-trying antecedents, and are smokers, drinkers and over and above cannabis use, are weekend stimulant-led poly drug users.

In Europe

Interestingly this basic profile resonates with descriptions from around Europe in respect of dance drug use being a key part of the young adult social scenes. The Calafat study (1998) confirms the importance of 'going out' with drugs although cannabis features more strongly in some European countries whereas stimulant drug use is less common. Studies around Europe predictably identify different rates of dance drug use. Countries like Germany and Denmark have far higher rates than say Finland or France. The Netherlands, whilst its youth population is generally far less drug involved than in the UK, does have a very comparable clubber–pay party scene.

One large-scale Dutch study based on describing several party venues and questioning 1,121 customers found that 16–21 was the dominant age group (40 per cent). These respondents were either studying or working and three-quarters lived at home. Half were regular party goers although with age the frequency of attendance fell and the 'elders' migrated to quieter, smaller venues, perhaps because three-quarters of the overall sample spent at least half of a very long night on the dance floor! The established 'gateways' via alcohol, tobacco and cannabis were found and with 81 per cent having taken ecstasy, 63 per cent amphetamines and three-quarters cannabis, again we find a very drug-experienced customer base. Less alcohol was consumed by these Dutch ravers and what was an educated, affluent sample were said to 'integrate their ecstasy and their everyday lives effectively' (Van de Wyngaart et al., 1998).

The dance drug users

We find the dance drug users amongst the clubbers and party goers. The clubbers are in turn socially located in the larger, young adult, 'going out' population who congregate mainly at weekends. Their chosen leisure locations are still linked to licensed venues both because the sale of alcohol sustains this sector of the leisure industry and because as a licit psycho-active drug, alcohol remains the most frequently consumed substance. Thus the drinkers and the drug users, who often drink as well, share the same scene.

This 'going out' population is made up of devotees from a wide variety of socio-economic backgrounds but with students and employed people being strongly represented. What distinguishes this overall population from their peers is the emphasis on the consumption of music, dancing, tobacco, alcohol and drugs. The dance drug users thus stand out from an already conspicuous lifestyle group by being extremely drug experienced. They are poly drug users, who routinely combine tobacco, alcohol and illicit drugs. Yet in turn they are distinguished and distinguishable from most problem drug users by social class, employment and education, criminality, frequency and quantity of use and drugs imbibed, although the rise in cocaine use may fray this bifurcation between addictive and less addictive drugs.

UK clubbers share much with their European 'time outers'. However, and whilst national profiles vary in respect of illicit drug use, the final point is salutary. European comparative studies show that the rates of dance drug use are *far higher* in the UK than elsewhere in Europe. Using comparative survey data numerous analyses reach the same conclusions. The most authoritative study of designer or synthetic drug use which compared ten EU countries utilised comparative national survey data. In respect of these drugs – amphetamines, LSD and ecstasy – the UK was far and away the league table topper having lifetime and past year rates over twice as high as the next highest placed country and over three times as high as the remainder (Griffiths et al., 1997). This is another reason why the British dance drug–clubber population is so important to study. It is one arena we must examine if we are to begin to understand why the UK has such an exceptionally drug-experienced population.

Pathways to dance drug use

There have been few attempts to explain how adolescents at say, 16, become regular clubbers and dance drug users by the time they're 20. Again we do not have sufficient research data to fully answer this question. However there are numerous clues from the Nineties research into adolescent and post-adolescent lifestyles which can begin to frame and explain this transition. Firstly we must recognise that journeying towards dance drug use is based on making and remaking drugs decisions through time and with life and leisure experience.

Cost-benefit drugs decision making

With the exception of one small study of mid-adolescents most of whom were non-drug triers (Shiner and Newburn, 1997), all the main qualitative studies of the 1990s have emphasised that British youth make rational cost-benefit assessments about becoming involved in recreational drug use and limiting or broadening their repertoires. Six studies undertaken independently and with different adolescent populations all identified this approach to decision making around cannabis (e.g. Coffield and Gofton, 1994) as opposed to trying more 'dangerous' substances (Young and Jones, 1997), or constructing boundaries and rules and learning to use a particular drug in 'sensible' ways (Hirst and McCamley-Finney, 1994; Hart and Hunt, 1997; Boys et al., 2000).

These studies based on interviews and discussion groups noted how a hierarchy of dangerousness was drawn up around which drugs were safe to try or use. Wholly consistent with the prevalence rates for different drugs across the 1990s, the consensus amongst the youth samples studied was that cannabis was benign whilst heroin and crack cocaine were simply never to be tried, being addictive drugs with dreadful reputations. Views on amphetamines, tranquillisers and LSD were more diverse. Ecstasy, because of its demonisation by the media during the mid-1990s, was seen as more dangerous by those who were mid-adolescents earlier in the decade. The risks and negatives in the assessment revolved around immediate health problems, being ill, having bad trips, comedowns, insomnia and getting caught. The benefits or gains were seen as distinctive to each drug depending on whether the main goals were to be mellow or relaxed, self-confident and sociable, energetic and alert or simply 'buzzing' or 'getting out of it'. This same assessment procedure was identified by Parker et al. (1998).

These studies also emphasise that most young people see drug use as fitting into their everyday conventional activities of studying, working, seeing friends, playing sport and so on. All these findings are broadly consistent with similar studies of young adults (Perri et al., 1997; Boys et al., 2000).

Drugs pathways to regular use

The second type of analysis involves longitudinal monitoring of young people's drug use across adolescence. However such studies are very expensive and unless extremely well resourced can suffer from attrition, particularly at 16 when half the UK youth population leave school. In this section we summarise the pathways analyses gleaned from two longitudinal studies of drugwise Nineties youth. We focus on the characteristics of the early entrants to the dance club–night club scene at around 16 to 18 years of age using both quantitative analysis and interview data from a sub sample of the cohorts followed across most of the 1990s (see Breeze et al. (forthcoming); Aldridge et al., 1999; Measham et al., 1998b; Parker et al., 1998).

The North West Longitudinal Study (see Parker et al., 1998) initially followed several hundred young people from when they were 14 (in 1991) until they were 18 using annual confidential self-report questionnaires and also interviews with 86 people when they were 17. This sample contained the archetypal 1990s' drugwise adolescents who are becoming the twentysomethings of the new post-millennial decade. At 18 (year five) with around 530 still in the sample, about a third had tried one or more of the dance drugs (amphetamines 33 per cent, poppers 35 per cent, ecstasy 20 per cent, cocaine 6 per cent). However, as we can see from Table 1.2, even from 14 (year one, 1991) we find early onset, with incidence growing annually. So well before any possible access to the club scene we find dance drug use. This said, the scale of initiation – for instance with ecstasy, amphetamines and cocaine – increases significantly at 17 and 18 (years four and five) as access to the going out–time out world becomes a reality.

Table 1.2   N.W. Longitudinal Study lifetime prevalence of illicit drug trying (age 14–18 incl)

	Year One (N = 776) %	Year Two (N = 752) %	Year Three (N = 523) %	Year Four (N = 536) %	Year Five (N = 529) %
Amphetamines	9.5	16.1	18.4	25.2	32.9
Amyl Nitrite	14.2	22.1	23.5	31.3	35.3
Cannabis	31.7	41.5	45.3	53.7	59.0
Cocaine	1.4	4.0	2.5	4.5	5.9
Heroin	0.4	2.5	0.6	0.6	0.6
LSD	13.3	25.3	24.5	26.7	28.0
Magic Mushrooms	9.9	12.4	9.8	9.5	8.5
Ecstasy	5.8	7.4	5.4	12.9	19.8
Solvents	11.9	13.2	9.9	10.3	9.5
Tranquillisers	1.2	4.7	1.5	3.9	4.5
At least one	36.3	47.3	50.7	57.3	64.3

A drugs status or pathways analysis was undertaken which showed that at 17 and 18 the sample was made up of four distinctive clusters: abstainers, former triers, current drug users and those in transition. *Abstainers* had never tried a drug and declared that they never intended to. They also held anti-drugs attitudes. *Former triers* whilst they had taken drugs in the past no longer did so and did not expect to do so again. *Current drug users* held pro-drug attitudes, used drugs currently and regularly and expected to continue to do so. Those *in transition* held fairly positive drug attitudes and whilst most had tried a drug this group did not consider themselves users of drugs. Most importantly however all those in transition expected to take or retake a drug in the future.

Those who had tried or were using the main dance drugs of poppers, amphet-amines, ecstasy and cocaine powder (far less available in 1996) were nearly all in the current users' group. By 18, 70 per cent of this current user group has past week drug use, had tried over four different drugs and expected to continue taking drugs. Only the in-transition group appeared to have the potential to produce dance drug users and it will be from this group that later onset of dance drug use, say during college and early career years, is likely to occur (see Parker et al., 1998).

Turning now to the other longitudinal 'drugs pathways' study based, thus far, on three annual surveys of about 1,300 13- to 15-year-olds and 1,300 15- to 17-year-olds, Table 1.3 highlights the under-eighteens dance drug experience of young people in two regions of Northern England in the late 1990s (see Egginton et al., 2001; Aldridge et al., 1999). We can see how in general as adolescence unfolds, illicit drugs become more and more available to young people with offer rates of amphetamines at over 40 per cent for the 15-year-olds and over 50 per cent for the 17-year-olds in 1998. We can also see that with amphetamines, the second most widely used street drug after cannabis, already 20 per cent of 17-year-olds have tried it and 13 per cent in the past year. Rates for ecstasy use are also clearly rising with age.

The regular drug users (Egginton et al., 2001) in this large longitudinal study again displayed the same antecedents as early risk takers, sensation seekers, early drinkers and smokers and drugs experimenters (Aldridge et al., 1998). However once again the equivalent of an in-transition or in this study potential user group was found. In other words amongst those who have tried drugs, over half of both age cohorts, we found up to half expect to try drugs again in the future (as well as 21–29 per cent who do not and 27 per cent who are more regular users already). It is going to be mainly from this potential user group that any later entrants to dance drug use emerge.

This repeating picture gives strong clues about who makes the early transition from adolescent drug trying to regular dance drug use. The dance drug users predominately come from the significant minority of adolescents who tend to be smokers, are regular drinkers and early illicit drug triers. They have distinguishable characteristics (Parker et al. 2001; Aldridge et al., 1998). They are probably joined by later 'entrants' in young adulthood who are likely to have the characteristics of the in-transition group defined earlier.

The catalyst or set and setting for the development of more regular dance drug use and the increases in incidence in post-adolescence is, to return to our key theme, going out and time out. From around the age of 17 access to weekend adventures in pubs, bars and clubs provides the pathway.

A small sub sample (n = 27) of the older cohort was interviewed annually three times between 1996 and 1998 (Breeze et al., 2001; Measham et al., 1998b). A remarkable consistency was found in the way 'time out' weekends quickly developed and impacted upon both drinkers who did and didn't take drugs. This social habit of going out in social networks to concerts, gigs, but especially circuit drinking in town, usually followed by a late night bar or 'younger' night club embraced young people with a range of drugs experience. For drugs abstainers who joined this time out world they experienced far more situations where drugs were available and used. For those with previous drugs experience they saw and heard far more about ecstasy and cocaine powder in particular.

Table 1.3   Northern Regions Study: Dance drug use before 18 years of age % (rounded)

Younger Cohort (13–15 years)	1996 (n = 1310)			1997 (n = 1461)			1998 (n = 1342)		
	Offered	Ever Tried	Past Year	Offered	Ever Tried	Past Year	Offered	Ever Tried	Past Year
Cannabis	24	15	12	41	26	21	62	42	37
Poppers	9	6	4	18	17	11	40	24	15
Amphetamines	12	5	4	22	9	6	41	17	13
LSD	11	5	4	20	8	5	32	11	8
Ecstasy	8	2	1	13	3	2	25	5	4
Cocaine	7	1	1	9	2	1	15	4	3

Older Cohort (15–17 years)	1996 (n = 1310)			1997 (n = 1461)			1998 (n = 1794)*		
	Offered	Ever Tried	Past Year	Offered	Ever Tried	Past Year	Offered	Ever Tried	Past Year
Cannabis	60	44	37	70	50	40	76	51	40
Poppers	32	19	13	48	28	16	44	23	8
Amphetamines	35	18	15	44	20	15	53	20	13
LSD	37	14	11	43	17	10	41	13	6
Ecstasy	26	6	5	36	10	8	45	11	8
Cocaine	10	2	1	12	2	1	20	3	3

* Subject to Attrition

For the abstainers to be in such social settings involved both tolerating others' drug use and having strategies to say no without acrimony. Some struggle:

... just different times when I've been around different people and they've shown me little bags of stuff or whatever they've got. It's too numerous to remember really. It seems to have got worse this year. I've been around it more and more. I'm sort of very passive about it, when I've been offered drugs I just think it's another knob head.

(Male, Abstainer, 17 years)

Others accommodate:

If I saw some I wouldn't gasp like I would before, because you see people all the time now who you know have been on them and you know have got them. My mates still take it [cannabis/amphetamines] and I don't know what they'll go into next. They say you start on cannabis and you go on to something bigger. I don't think they will but I don't know.

(Male, Abstainer, 17 years)

Others, in time, become drug involved themselves, emphasising the key point that initiation into and extensions of drugs experience continues right across adolescence, into the twenties and beyond:

So I thought I've have cider this week. We were watching my friend in the band in Bradford. Then we went back to my friend's ... and had a few drinks there and then we went into town. It didn't even cross my mind to do it, but I was having a really good night and I thought right ... Sal ran into the toilets and went 'Tina, Tina come here.' I went in and she started taking speed. She said 'Do you want some? I promise I won't give you enough to make you ill. I'll give you a tiny bit.' So I took it.

(Female, Initiate, 17 years)

The very first time I had a full pill to myself was the very first night I went out clubbing. I remember I threw up and after I threw up I felt amazing. I felt brilliant. I must have introduced myself to everyone in the club that night.

(Female, Poly Drug User, 16 years)

Conclusion

The UK has one of the most drug-involved populations amongst post-industri-alised societies. It now has proportionately as many young drug takers as the States, a far larger dance drug scene and heads the European league table for recreational drug use.

This unprecedented growth in drug use may have had its roots in the 1970s and 1980s but manifested itself during the 1990s. Availability of most street drugs is routine for the majority of today's young Britons. By the end of ado-lescence, accepting regional differences, between 50 and 65 per cent will have tried illicit drugs and 20–25 per cent will be occasional to regular users. Whilst cannabis defines youthful recreational drug use in the UK, we now have a small but significant minority who are dance drug users. The use of amphetamines, ecstasy, and increasingly, cocaine have become part of their poly drug use which also includes alcohol. They have blurred the licit and the illicit. This process is most noticeable in the going out–time out scene where alcohol remains a central drug. We have argued elsewhere that all these changes indicate the process of normalisation of recreational drug use, particularly in late and post-adolescence. We have also argued that for normalisation to be claimed we need to find 'sensible' recreational drug use, despite its illegality, acknowledged and tolerated by non-drug users or ex-drug triers. This social accommodation begins in mid-adolescence but seems to increase with age and life experience. One key reason for this is that the *majority* of today's young adults have taken drugs and live unscathed to tell the tale. Another is that whilst there will always be a minority in any age cohort who hold strong 'anti' views about something, be it smoking or illegal drug use, it does seem that non-drug users who are outgoing come to accept that those around them may take drugs. Because in the main this behaviour is benign in respect of friendships, informal parties, romantic relationships, socialising and dancing, then there is accommodation and tolerance.

What we do not yet know is whether these processes identified in late and post-adolescent populations will carry over into adulthood as 1990s drugwise youth become twentysomething citizens in the new decade. Will recreational drug use rates grow amongst younger adults as they have amongst adolescents? Will the behaviour of some adults in respect of drugs be acceptable to their peers or will more conservative, conventional attitudes prevail? Although there are signs of recreational drug use growing amongst young adults and indeed of greater tolerance by non-users, we will need to wait for several years before we can fully answer this question. A key indicator will be whether recent drug use grows amongst the 25 to 30 age group, as it is doing in the 19 to 24, whereby the traditional 'settling down' period is delayed as drug use is sustained both by new cultural acceptance combined with longer transitions to full citizenship and 'responsibility'. This drug use will also need to remain in social and semi-public settings. If it becomes covert, privatised and stigmatised then we have seen the limits of normalisation. All this is important to provide the backcloth to understanding the clubbers. They are, even by UK standards, 'excessive' alcohol and drugs consumers. Whilst perhaps half the post-adolescent–young adult population go out for 'time out' and most will have tried drugs, the regular dance drug users are a minority of this sector. In exploring dance drug use in the British club scene we are thus connecting with one of the most drug-experienced populations 'available' outside problem drug-user populations (which revolve around heroin or crack cocaine). The clubbers are at the most serious end of recreational drug use in a country with an exceptionally high rate of drug involvement. Both their lifetime and recent rates of taking cannabis, amphetamines, poppers, LSD, ecstasy and cocaine are many times higher than those found in the overall adolescent and adult populations.

We have offered one possible explanation as to how the clubbers develop these drugs profiles so quickly and so distinctively. We have argued that rather than coming from delinquent or deviant backgrounds (but see Hammersley et al., 1999) they are in fact mostly fairly conventional adolescents except in their tendency to be early risk takers, sensation seekers and socially outgoing. They share these characteristics with a significant minority of the population who in previous generations, as we shall see in the next chapter, also valued going out and time out but who were largely limited to alcohol as the chemical aid.

Today's going out–time out consumers have ready access to illegal chemical assistance and a minority take up dance drug use. We have suggested that the migratory population to the dance club and dance drugs is primarily made up of young people who are outgoing and utilise numerous substances including alcohol and tobacco to stimulate or self-medicate. They are introduced to all this through connecting, from around the age of 17, with the commercial, time out leisure world. Once in this social space of dance clubs, circuit bar drinking, café bar nights and 'under 21s' clubs, they quickly hear, see and learn more about amphetamines, ecstasy and cocaine, thereby furthering their drugs apprenticeships. However this is not the only migratory route.

Some young people who remained far more conforming in adolescence join the dance club and night club later, often via college lifestyles or new friendship patterns. This is consistent with the overall socio-economic profile of the clubbers. All this is socialisation through socialising.

We do not really understand why the UK drugs landscape is as it is and why British society should be the primary site for such social transformation compared with other similar countries. The parallel but slightly more muted process under way amongst Europe's going out populations is primarily explained through post-modernity – consumption of leisure perspectives. These are undoubtedly crucial but they do not fully explain the UK's unique drugs status.

Whilst we will not create a wholly satisfactory explanation for the UK's unique drugs status without detailed comparative historical and cultural studies, in the next chapter we turn our attention to current debates surrounding the cultural context for dance drug use. Any study of current British dance drug use is not complete without an understanding of the distinctiveness of the British cultural context and the significance of dance club culture. We offer an overview of developments in British dancing and clubbing, musical genres and evolving venues through a consideration of the significance of social divisions and difference to club culture. There is an intensity and integrity to the development of clubbing in Britain from the post-war period right through to the 'decade of dance' and the new millennium which helps us understand why dance drugs and dance clubs are so intimately related and why 'time out' weekends are so important.

2 Identity and Location in Clubland: Gender, Class, Race, Sexual Orientation and Club Culture

INTRODUCTION

The last chapter focused on the current debate, predominantly in the fields of criminology, social policy and the addictions, surrounding dance *drugs*. This chapter considers the current debate surrounding dance *clubs*, which has predominantly occurred within cultural studies, cultural criminology, music journalism and the popular press.[1] Although there is a long history of social dancing and of clubs, we will look here at dance clubs as a specific leisure location. The dance club has been a key social space for British youth since the post-war era and yet the 'decade of dance' at the end of the twentieth century was seen by many academic and popular commentators as a new cultural phenomenon. This chapter will consider the similarities and distinctions between dancing and clubbing in the 1990s and earlier decades, alongside an exploration of the identity of clubbers, covering issues of gender, race, socio-economic class and sexual orientation in the dance club scene.

WAVES OF RAVE

Before doing this, however, we will briefly discuss the term the 'decade of dance' and consider the phases within it. The 'decade of dance' is usually used to refer to the period 1988–98. In part the 'decade of dance' was a term coined in the mid-1990s, in anticipation of the marketing opportunities in 1998, and thus was a promotions strategy for the plethora of compilation music albums, books and journal articles with a retrospective consideration of the rave and dance club scene. As it was widely accepted that the rave scene broke out in 1988 (e.g. Anthony, 1998), 1998 then became a useful focus point for the publication of these musical and literary retrospectives. The term was also picked up by clubbers as well, however, in celebration of the survival of dance culture in the face of apparent attempts to suppress it by the authorities (McDermott, 1993; Measham et al., 1998a). The enormous changes within club culture – the diversification and fragmentation from a single underground rave scene into a myriad of sub-

19

genres – belies the implications of stability and coherence in the notion the 'decade of dance'. Indeed Garratt suggests that even as early as 1990 there was no one dance club 'scene' as such:

> By 1990, it was no longer possible to talk of one single 'scene', but far from weakening the growing club culture, this fragmentation only served to make it stronger. As everyone took the basic ingredients and adapted them to their own needs, backgrounds, tastes and drugs of choice, the music began to mutate endlessly, splitting off into interlinked scenes and sub-cultures that continue to influence and feed back into each other in the most unexpected ways. (1998, pp. 258–9)

Within this overall evolution of the rave and dance club scene from its origins through to the present, commentators such as Reynolds (1998) and Henderson (1993a) have identified three main phases:

(i)   1988–89: The first wave – ACID HOUSE. The original underground, in pockets around the country.

(ii) 1990–92: The second wave – RAVE. The peak: popular, widespread, national, but yet to be systematically commercially exploited.

(iii) 1993 onwards: The third wave – DANCE. Commercial, fragmenting into sub-genres, growing problems of policing, licensing, and criminal involvement. As we shall see later in this chapter, this period is sometimes characterised as the UK rave scene turned from dream to nightmare. (For a more detailed history of the developments within the rave and dance scene see Collin and Godfrey, 1997, Garratt, 1998, and Reynolds, 1998.)

The rest of this chapter will discuss firstly, the similarities between dance club culture and previous British youth cultures, then secondly, the ways in which the demographic profile of clubbers was dissimilar to previous youth cultures.

THE DANCE GOES ON: SIMILARITIES BETWEEN DANCE CLUB CULTURE IN THE 1990S AND PREVIOUS YOUTH CULTURES

Although a distinctive British and American youth culture is seen as originating in the 1940s post-war era, the links between British youth, dancing, leisure and indeed drugs can be traced back to another post-war era. Newspaper records have assisted in the identification of a media 'moral panic' surrounding young people's dancing and drug use in the 1920s not dissimilar to forthcoming generations (Pearson, 1983; Kohn, 1992). Small numbers of young people attended jazz clubs in the West End of London, consumed cocaine and danced for hours.

From the 1950s and 1960s, Top Rank and Mecca ballrooms popularised dance halls in cities across the country. After a lull in the early 1970s which led to suggestions that we had witnessed the death of mass dances by 1976 (Mungham, 1976), the dance hall continued in the form of 1970s discotheques, 1980s night clubs, and 1990s dance clubs. Attending late-night clubs to drink, dance and socialise has been a more or less central part of the weekend for considerable numbers of young people for decades. Whilst the styles of popular music, clothes and dance steps changed, alongside the styles of lighting, interior design and sound systems, in many British cities these developments have occurred within the same spaces – the very same architectural structures – across the years. The names changed, but for many clubs the function stayed the same.

Classic studies within criminology and the sociology of deviance in the 1960s and 1970s charted youth subcultures and the centrality of clothes, music and Saturday night dancing as a part of identity politics, of working-class (male) youthful rebellion against middle-class/adult values through their development of a distinct subcultural style (Hall and Jefferson, 1976; Mungham and Pearson, 1976). As Hebdige has noted, 'the cycle leading from opposition to defusion, from resistance to incorporation encloses each successive subculture' (1979, p. 100).

The lack of studies focussing specifically on the dance hall as a social setting and dancing as a working-class, leisure-time pursuit have been noted, for example, by Sherlock (1993), Mungham (1976), and Rust (1969). In the 1970s Mungham noted the lack of research on dancing and dance halls and felt that 'the neglect of the dance sits strangely at odds with the fact of its evident popularity among working class youth' (1976, p. 85). His comment still resonates today.

The use of alcohol and/or illicit drugs has also been discussed as a distinguishing feature of specific British youth subcultures from the cocaine girls of the 1920s (Kohn, 1992, 1997) to the amphetamine-consuming mods of the 1960s (Cohen, 1972; Hebdige, 1976a) and the punks and skinheads of the 1970s (Hebdige, 1979; Moore, 1994). In many respects, therefore, there was a clear lineage in twentieth-century Britain from these previous dance music/club subcultures to the ecstasy-fuelled rave culture of the 1990s (Newcombe, 1991; Gilman, 1994; Collin and Godfrey, 1997). 'Raving' can be seen as the latest in a long line of working-class youth cultures whose key component is 'living for the weekend' and clubbing in particular. The ups and downs of 'the working-class weekender life cycle of drudgery, anticipation and explosive release' (Reynolds, 1997, p. 110), illustrated in films such as *Quadrophenia* (about 1960s mods) and *Human Traffic* (about 1990s dance clubbers), have changed little since the 1950s. The growth of post-war working-class leisure will be discussed later in this chapter but here we outline the case for *continuity* in youth cultures, in part reflecting the continuity in the cycles, structure and economic relations, if not the content, of work and leisure in post-war Britain.

Historically, British public houses have been seen as social spaces predominantly occupied by working-class men and for quieter weekday drinking, whereas dance halls and night clubs have been a highlight of female and male weekend leisure, an opportunity for dancing, heavy drinking and romantic/sexual liaisons (Harrison, 1971; Mungham, 1976; Hey, 1986; Plant, 1997). This historical importance of clubs to youth culture has related in part to the economic costs of cubic space in Britain and in part to the physical and social geography of youth. Without cars to cruise in, without warm and dry weather most of the year to sit outside in, without large houses for privacy and entertaining guests, without cheap or free local phone calls, with few affordable evening eating venues, with indoor shopping malls a relatively recent phenomenon, pubs and night clubs have traditionally been key social spaces for working-class British young adults, by comparison with Europe or North America. Thornton (1995) has noted that the primacy of clubs might be unique to Britain and contrasts British youth with American youth, who have had relatively larger houses, access to free local phone calls, relatively cheaper evening eating venues (such as diners and fast food outlets), indoor malls in abundance and a greater emphasis on car ownership. All these have enabled American youth to carve out a social space and obtain a degree of privacy from parents and other adults in which to conduct friendships and romantic/sexual relationships. In many ways, Thornton suggests, the American car and the British club are analogous social spaces.

Having considered cultural continuities we will now consider the *distinctions* of dance. It should be noted, however, that whether or not current dance club culture is considered a break with the past, both analyses assume a linear development of youth cultures. A critique of this concept of linear youth cultures in post-war Britain is provided by Redhead. Redhead prefers instead the concept of cycles and recycling, combinations and recombinations, whereby 'the cyclical motion is embedded in pop's genealogy' (1990, p. 25). As we reach the end of the century, Redhead suggests that in post-modern debates fixed notions of youth culture, subculture and deviance have been replaced by a fluidity and flexibility around counter cultures, lifestyles, identities, the mass media and mass markets. With his play on the term 'counter culture', Redhead suggests that '"Counter cultures" is now more resonant of shopping and consumption rather than resistance and deviance' (1990, p. 90).

KEY DISTINCTIONS IN THE 'DECADE OF DANCE': CHARACTERISTICS OF CLUBBERS IN 1990S BRITISH DANCE CLUB CULTURE

A key debate in relation to the 'decade of dance' is its qualitative and quantitative significance. Was this another in a long line of British youth (sub)cultures, or was there something unique about it, in terms of scale (moving from sub-cultural to mainstream involvement), participation and/or in terms of its cultural significance?

Writings on rave include both academic and popular perspectives. Although academic studies on the subject of 1990s rave and dance culture are starting to filter through to publication, the earliest and most influential writers have been popular commentators and music journalists involved in the dance scene, as well as clubbers themselves. The academic studies of dance clubs are multi-disciplinary, although clustered under the umbrella of cultural studies, and many of them are by students and younger academics who have direct connections with the dance club scene (for example, see Newcombe, 1991, 1992a, 1992b; Redhead, 1993; Thornton, 1995).There has also been a wave of rave fiction alongside the histories of rave. (Best known of these writers of fiction, 'the poet laureate of the chemical generation' [*The Face*], is Welsh, 1993, 1994, 1995, 1996. See also Champion, 1997.) The problems in writing about the rave and dance scene, however, are threefold. Firstly does a distinct rave/dance culture as such exist which can be identified and discussed? Secondly, as noted by Reynolds, if one assumes that there is a distinct dance culture, does the very nature of this phenomenon (sensation-based, experiential) defy attempts at verbal expression? In Reynolds' view writings on rave have tried, struggled and mostly failed to express those experiences shared by millions of ravers and therefore he asks:

So how do you write the history of a culture that is fundamentally amnesiac and non-verbal? ... Where rock relates an experience ... rave *constructs* an experience. Bypassing interpretation, the listener is hurled into a vortex of heightened sensations, abstract emotions and artificial energies. ... Rave provokes the question: is it possible to base a culture around sensations rather than truths, fascination rather than meaning? (1998, p. xix)

And thirdly, if one assumes a distinct dance culture does exist and even if it is possible to capture and represent it in words, do we want to, politically? This relates to a point made by Sharma et al. regarding black and Asian dance culture being an object of knowledge for academic consumption and an object of middle-class liberals' enduring fascination with 'Otherness', other cultures and exotica (1996). Academic inquisitiveness and academic consumption of black youth cultures, of the 'Other' is seen by Sharma et al. to have 'close ideological connections with the disciplines of command that police inner-urban neighbourhoods ... ' (Sharma et al., 1996, p. 2).

They suggest that interest in black and working-class dance music youth cultures cannot be divorced from a climate of continuing socio-economic inequalities where prioritisation is given to the policing of the inner city, of black and working-class youth, resulting in amongst other things the closing down of black/dance clubs.[2] Any exploration of dance club culture such as this chapter must, therefore, acknowledge this political context and 'not reduce popular culture to the scrutinized Other' (Sharma et al., 1996, p. 3). Hebdige develops the role of the scrutinising academic further in the concluding remarks to his exploration of British punk subculture, where he suggests that it is the academic rather than the subject of study, who is the outsider, the 'Other':

> ... we, the sociologists and interested straights, threaten to kill with kindness the forms which we seek to elucidate. ... to get the point is, in a way, to miss the point. ... We are in society but not inside it, producing analyses of popular culture which are themselves anything but popular. (Hebdige, 1979, pp. 139–40)

This question of perspective is central to the theme of this chapter: culture and society. Academic explorations of British working-class leisure since the nineteenth century have considered issues of regulation and social control, with one of the recurrent themes for both historians and contemporary commentators being the distinctions between the 'respectable' working class and the 'rough' working class or casual residuum (Stedman Jones, 1971). Attempts have been made to channel 'respectable' working-class leisure pursuits through public parks, libraries, museums, churches, restricted pub opening hours and the temperance movement. Simultaneously the 'rougher' elements of pre-industrial and industrial popular culture evident in heavy drinking (particularly in gin palaces), street gambling, animal fighting, traditional fairs, festivals and races have been suppressed, criminalised and in many cases died out (Stedman Jones, 1983). Even within the dance hall, attempts have been made to distinguish between the 'rough' and 'respectable' working class, as Mungham has noted (1976).

Having considered some concerns which have been raised regarding any attempt to represent dance club culture in textual form, we will look at the spiritual and political significance of the dance scene before outlining some of the key characteristics in the demographic profile of clubbers.

Spiritual and political significance

A key feature of the rave/dance scene was its emphasis on utopianism. Whilst this makes the early 1990s rave movement in many ways spiritually closer to the 1960s hippie subculture with its 'luv'd up' vibe, it clearly demarcates it from the main British post-war youth subcultures of teds, mods, punks, skinheads, new romantics, goths, heavy rockers, grunge and indie. This utopian ideal of peace, love and positivity was in evidence in the first two waves of rave before its transmutation into the mainstream commercial dance scene. (Remnants of the 'peace, love and unity' of the early rave scene are still recognisable in the predominantly young, white and provincial 'happy hardcore' scene, however, which developed after the split in the hardcore rave scene in 1993. For more details on hardcore, gabba and funcore, see Reynolds, 1998, Chapter 11.) In interviews, commentaries and reviews from the earliest warehouse parties and raves through to the 'decade of dance' retrospectives, clubbers spoke of a feeling of unity with other clubbers, of euphoria or 'ecstasy' in clubland, of a spiritual and collective bonding which was absent from mainstream night clubs. As the following two quotes from clubbers show, this was true both for small inner-city Northern clubs:

> Everyone was dancing – not like in the alternative clubs we were used to, get up and have a groove to a song or two you liked and sit down again, but going for it big time: dancing for five or six hours, tops off, sweating like fuck ... and everyone with these big pool-ball eyes, huge grins, complete strangers coming up to you, 'Where ya from? What y'on? Y'having a good night?' No one wanted a battle. No one was pissed and falling all over you. All anyone wanted to do was dance. (Russell David, quoted in Harrison, 1998, p. 2)

And for large-scale outdoor Southern dance festivals:

> ... all around you were people who at that moment were thinking like you; had the same objectives as you; people who in the 'real world' you might not give the time of day but who would look out for you here; who you'd pass in the street without a glance but who were like family now; who had sober and responsible jobs and whole other lives and identities that at that time *didn't matter* because you were all here, in this place, with each other, to dance. (Anon, talking about Tribal Gathering, quoted in Harrison, 1998, p. 12)

Spiritual: ecstatic states

It has been suggested that the rave/dance club scene was just another example of hedonistic, risk-taking youth (Plant and Plant, 1992). Even the most mystical explanations of the dance scene could be interpreted as rationalisations or spiritualisations of the bottom-line centrality of getting intoxicated on illicit dance drugs. After all, 'losing it' and 'altered states' may refer to higher levels of consciousness but in youthful terminology they also refer to excessive levels of intoxication through psycho-active drug use (Reynolds, 1998).

Other commentators and researchers, however, have noted the spiritual undertones of the rave/dance phenomenon evident in social behaviour and etiquette within dance clubs. This can be placed within the wider historical context of the 'decade of dance'. Over the course of the twentieth century, there has been declining participation in religious and church services, declining trade union activism and fewer political rallies and marches, resulting in few situations

where thousands of like-minded people gather together to witness or participate in an event. This leaves sports events, dance clubs and royal weddings and
funerals to provide some of the only opportunities for collective social or spiritual
bonding. Furthermore, the timing of this 'end-of-century' party has been linked
with New Age spirituality, millennial cults and *fin de siècle* fears.

There was a quasi-religious tone to the awe with which some people described
their conversion to the rave/dance scene. For example, at Shoom, one of the
very first Ibiza-inspired, Balearic house clubs which opened in November 1987,
'people were walking round like they'd found Christianity' (Jak, quoted in
Garratt, 1998, p. 114). Newcombe, one of the earliest academic researchers of the
British rave phenomenon, has noted the quasi-religious experience of dance
clubs in his studies. The minimal lyrics and repetitive chants of much dance
music, for example, have been likened to religious mantras. DJs, MCs and
promoters were revered as cultural heroes, particularly the DJs whose presence
up on stage in front of the crowds has been likened to a priest at a church altar
with the congregation spread out before them:

> ... DJs are the high priests and priestesses of the rave ceremony, responding
> to the mood of the crowd, with their mixing desks symbolising the altar (the
> only direction towards which ravers consistently face is the DJ box).
> (Newcombe, 1992b, p. 5)

Lewis has also noted the 'divine status' of 'sacred persons' such as DJs, dance
party promoters and even drug dealers in the Sydney gay dance party scene
(1994).

Rather than simply quasi-religious symbols, the deeper spiritual significance
of dance parties has been emphasised by some commentators. Cross-culturally,
the modern dance party scene has been likened to the '3D' tribal rituals of many
pre-industrial societies where dance, drugs and drums are used in group settings
with the aim of creating a collective state of altered consciousness or 'archaic consciousness' (McKenna, 1992). This cyberdelic, New Age, trance-dance spirituality,
particularly in evidence in the San Francisco rave scene of the early 1990s,
developed into a specific sub-genre of rave music called ambient which continues
in the form of groups such as the Orb, for example. In Britain too, Newcombe
noted that

> the ecstatic state sought and achieved by ravers is arguably the expression of
> a primal urge for group revelry and carnival. ... the ancient human instinct
> to celebrate existence and alter awareness by group dancing and drug taking
> ... (Newcombe, 1991, p. 5)

This essentialist, ahistoric, universalising of the spirituality of dance culture has been criticised elsewhere for denying the ethnically-specific nature of these influences. Sharma et al. ask: 'Why is it that writings about Techno and Rave erase their Black antecedents and continued Black influence through deracialized accounts of trance dance tribalism and the shamanic disappearance of the body?' (Sharma et al., 1996, p. 6).

Rietveld has also suggested that the central meaning of the dance subculture was this loss of self in the ritual of the dance and that 'no meaning could be found other than pure escape' (1993, p. 43). She notes that rave culture was not overtly rebellious and that it did not attempt to challenge mainstream culture:

Rather than creating a spectacle of resistance ... the rave offered ... a temporary escapist disappearance like the weekend or holiday. ... there was an offensive against the established order by negating its rationale, through the surrender to a void. A Dionysian[3] ritual of dance and hedonism evolved, whereby the established 'self' was undone. (Rietveld, 1993, p. 58)

This was the dance in which to forget, to loose oneself; this was the Dionysian ritual of obliteration, of disappearance. (Rietveld, 1993, p. 63)

It is not just the ritual of the dance which provides the rave/dance scene with its spiritual significance, however. It is the whole club experience:

... comparing a rave to a disco would be like comparing New Year's Eve celebrations to having a quiet drink in the local pub. The unique setting of raves is an essential component to spark off the orgasmic 'trance dance' atmosphere sought by ravers ... (Newcombe, 1991, p. 16)

Political: hedonism in hard times[4]

The political aspects of the 'decade of dance' are equally open to debate. As we have seen above, most writers on the 'decade of dance' have mentioned the lack of explicit political aims or beliefs. It was considered hedonistic rather than political, a celebration rather than a protest. In Kohn's discussion of ravers, he recognises a lack of political radicalism:

Their radicalism is basically apolitical, concerned with inner perceptual states and the pursuit of sensations of collective intimacy. They have no pretensions to changing the world. (Kohn, 1997, p. 140)

However, by its very existence, the underground acid house and rave scene in its early inception could be considered an attempt by British youth to carve out a dance culture without State sanction or regulation, and without commercial involvement or institutional surveillance. If not overtly political in organisation or aims, there were elements of the dance culture which did have political significance, although this was not necessarily recognised by participants at the time. For example, the early acid house style of 'baggy' clothes was eulogised in the Happy Mondays' song 'Loose Fit' on their 1990 album *Pills 'n' Thrills and Bellyaches*, 'Ryder's manifesto of baggy bad taste and spiritual laissez-faire' (Reynolds, 1998, p. 93). The 'baggy' look was seen as a rejection of the 1980s 'yuppie' designer decade, dressing down to go out clubbing, rather than dressing up. Involving relaxed, functional, colourful and cheap sportswear and casualwear drawing on late 1960s hippie clothes for inspiration, it was an anti-fashion statement which emphasised the precedence of dancing over appearance:

> The Me Generation has been replaced by the We Generation ... It's a swift and street-level reaction against the self-consciousness of the 'cool' designer Eighties. (Garratt and Baker, 1989, pp. 106–7)

DJ and Hacienda regular Justin Robertson more explicitly linked the early rave scene to the economic and political climate of the late 1980s:

> The economic situation was so appalling for most people, and we all felt relieved that here was something we could be *part* of, rather than just watch the country go down the pan. It was a release valve, a reaction against yuppies and go-getter Thatcherite politics. (Justin Robertson, quoted in Garratt, 1998, p. 204)

Hills, a music journalist, suggested that dance club culture was not just a reaction to the economic and political climate, but that clubland itself provided one of the few communities in 1990s Britain:

> After 12 years of Conservative government our society has become disparate, cocooned and cold. One of the few communities that remains today is that of the networks built up around clubs and drugs. However flawed and fake they may be they exist, and provide one of the few support systems some people have. (Hills, 1993, p. 143)

The widespread consumption of dance drugs and mass mobilisation at dance events in themselves meant that youth resistance through style had a new edge. Attendance at dance events could involve a direct rebellion against British legislation and policing, leading to cat-and-mouse tactics between police and clubbers, promoters and licensing authorities throughout the 'decade of dance'. It is interesting to note that in the 1990s it was dance music in contrast to rock music which was seen as the threat to society. Dance club culture was clearly perceived by the authorities as a political threat, needing prompt political action and resulting in six key legislative changes alongside further policing initiatives (Garratt and Taggart, 1990; Measham et al., 1998a). Historically Garratt locates radical/protest rock music in times of affluence, whereas dance club culture thrives in hard times:

> When times get tougher, people tend to escape down the rabbit hole, ... past the doorman, down the corridor and into wonderland. And survival, taking pleasure at a time when misery is all that's on offer, can surely be a political act in itself. Overwhelmingly, the acid house and rave scenes were about a generation denied a place in society as a whole creating a space in which they could express themselves. (Garratt, 1998, p. 321)

But can a culture be both escapist and political? Can the celebration of sensations have any deeper political significance? These questions of political sig-nificance – whether dance culture is political rebellion or political indifference, nihilistic escapism or collective expression – are the very questions which absorb current debate on youth cultures (Redhead, 1990). Whilst Rietveld sees dance culture as a break with the established order, she suggests there was no political significance to this escapism because no alternative order was proposed. As a participant in the dance club scene, however, Reynolds in contrast personally embraces both escapist and political interpretations in his own experiences:

> ... despite its ostensibly escapist nature, rave has actually politicized me, made me think harder about questions of class, race, gender, technology. Mostly devoid of lyrics and almost never overtly political, rave music – like dub reggae and hip hop – uses sound and rhythm to construct psychic landscapes of exile and utopia. ... the utopian/dystopian dialectic ... (Reynolds, 1998, p. xx).

One aspect of being lost in oneself and one's dancing was the idea of making one's own entertainment on the dance floor, rather than waiting to be enter-tained. This attitude was evident in hardcore dance magazines like *Eternity* and *To The Core*. Reynolds has noted that in these, unlike more commercially successful, cross-genre, mass-circulation dance magazines like *Mixmag* and *Muzik*, it was the audience who was the predominant feature of club reviews rather than the DJs, singers and recording artists. If anyone, it was the ravers who were the stars.

And what was the longer-term significance of the 'decade of dance'? Was all the utopian energy diffused on the dance floor, or did it spread into everyday life? And if it did, for how long did it last? Perhaps the fact that it came to nothing, politically, is an indication of the priority of pleasure-seeking over politics for its participants. But how could the mass mobilisation of thousands of young people across the nation, taking psycho-active drugs, defying attempts at regulation, sometimes directly confronting the police, have no longer-term significance? For those who participated, it *felt at the time* like there was great political potential in these gatherings and perhaps this was its significance: the direct personal experience of the power and potential of collective mobilisation, of being a part of a community, regardless of its form or direction. Garratt reaches a similar, simpler conclusion about the meaning of club culture:

> All of the theory in the world can't explain what it's like to be there, in the middle of the floor, when a night takes off. To dance so hard you forget yourself, you lose track of time, you feel that the music, the crowd, the building itself is all one living organism, of which you are just a tiny part. Perhaps, in the end, all it really comes down to is that feeling. We did it because it was fun. And many of us had the time of our lives. (Garratt, 1998, p. 322)

Throughout the writings on dance culture, many of them by academics and music journalists with some empathy or involvement in the dance scene, there is a tension between pleasure and politics, in the search for political meaning. This echoes academic debates during the 1970s about the significance of earlier British youth subcultures which had leisure as their main focus, and the limitations of a leisure-based, commodity-based subculture (Hall and Jefferson, 1976). McRobbie, however, sees this search for political significance as unsatisfactory, in both the escapism versus opposition debate outlined above and in the abstract theorising of certain academics. She suggests a new line of analysis which considers the political significance of the widening employment opportunities in the dance music industry through the democratisation of dance music production. Currently, the culture and technology industries are two of the boom British industries of the millennium. This has allowed an offshoot, the youth culture/dance music industry, to become the new 'job-creation scheme' for working-class young men, and to a lesser extent young women, with few qualifications but plentiful (self-taught) technical skills and experience (McRobbie, 1999, p. 41). Employment in the youth culture industry offers escape; it is an updating of the rags-to-riches story of the boxer/footballer/rock star on an unprecedented and currently unknown scale but with the emphasis on skills rather than stars.

McRobbie advocates a more conventional line of political analysis to be applied to the culture industry focussing in particular on employment. She calls for further research on the socio-economic significance of labour market expansion in the dance music industry, the scale of job creation, employment rights, pay levels, career development, and wider issues such as the tensions between creativity and commercial interests. Some of the issues surrounding the democratisation of dance music will be considered further in the next section.

Demographic profile of clubbers

As discussed above, persuasive arguments have been made that the 'decade of dance' resulted in the democratisation of dance music, both in terms of participation and production. But what was the composition of this new influx? Was it from across all sections of society or was it more specifically located? The following section will consider issues of gender, socio-economic class, race and sexual orientation in relation to dance club culture.

Gender: dancing for themselves

There is a consensus on one key characteristic of the rave/dance club scene. The differently gendered ambience of 1990s clubs as social spaces – with women's prominent presence in them since the first wave of rave – has been one of the main distinctions of 1990s club culture compared with the composition of previous youth cultures. This is despite the many ways in which the dance music and leisure industries are traditionally gendered. We note the existence of a sexual division of labour, vertical and horizontal occupational segregation, lack of equal pay and lack of equal opportunities in the dance and leisure industries, for example, among DJs, MCs, promoters, producers, management, security staff and bar staff. There also exists a sexual division of labour amongst the peripheral protagonists of club culture, for example, organised criminals, those supplying illegal drugs[5] and duty-free alcohol, 'protection' workers, and so on. Henderson describes young women involved in the early 1990s rave scene as 'predominantly consumers of the culture, not its producers' (1999, p. 42), to which we would add that by the time of the commercialisation of dance culture in the late 1990s women were also its employees (in certain occupational categories) rather than its entrepreneurs.

Having noted the gendered nature of the dance music and leisure industries in terms of employment as well as production, and the informal economy as well as the formal economy, the rest of this section will now consider the ways in which gender interaction and the presence of women in dance clubs as *consumers* of club culture diverged from previous British youth cultures. Gender interaction in dance clubs was notably different from both previous youth cultures and also contemporary 'ordinary' night clubs because of two key inter-related factors: the prioritising of dancing above romantic/sexual encounters for both women and men, and the pharmacological/perceived effects of the consumption of dance drugs by the majority of clubbers. Each of these factors will now be considered.

Dancing

Dance as a generic activitiy is a form of (usually) non-verbal communication which reflects social relations in wider society and also reflects changes in the relationship between the sexes. As 'one of the earliest recorded forms of human behaviour' and 'a critical medium of human communication' (Hanna, 1988, p. 241), dance can provide a form of expression and release from the fluidity and change experienced in wider society. It can be argued that gender divisions and relationships are currently in some limited forms of transition in society, alongside which the social and sexual construction of self is more fluid. It has been suggested that some current forms of dance reflect this, symbolising an era of individualism, identity awareness and sensual rather than sexual pleasure in the wake of the HIV/AIDS pandemic (e.g. Lewis, 1994).

Aside from reflecting and reinforcing gender divisions in current society, dance also has the capacity to evaluate and challenge society's gendered activities, and the patterns of mating, power and dominance within them. Hanna's cross-cultural study of dance, gender and sexuality shows how dance as a generic activity is an inherently sexual art form through which women and men can both express and question sexual identity and gender roles. Although she comes to focus predominantly on theatrical dance in her book, Hanna also considers social and ritual dance and the potential power of each to challenge and change gender norms:

> ... expressive forms, such as dance, perpetuate the pervading ideology of gender; at other times they impugn and undermine it. Culture ... has trans-formative potential and operative dialectical processes. Change of ideas is rarely abrupt and absolute; under the veneer of transformation lies a mass of tradition. (1988, p. 242)

Hanna suggests that both sexes are able to transgress dominant society's norms, including gender norms, using certain dance techniques. For theatrical dance these include:

> ... role reversals, gender blurring, and equal opportunity. Images are safe arenas to deal with anxieties and curiosity. Dances with images that deviate from the accepted societal norm may well help alter the status quo. (1988, p. 246)

Historically, modern dance developed in antithesis to classical dance at the turn of the century: both as a demand by women for freedom from the con-straints of Victorian society and male-dominated ballet, and as an expression of the changing position of women in the Western world in the 1900s (Hanna, 1988). Throughout the first half of the twentieth century modern social dancing continued to consist of the pairing of opposite sex couples. By the 1960s the growing popularity of individual, unpartnered, free-style modern social dancing in dance halls and night clubs was evident, centring around women dancing and men watching (and drinking) earlier in the evening, then women and men pairing up later in the evening.

Modern social dance, as with other group behaviour within post-war British youth cultures, has been seen as an expression of generational conflict and sub-cultural style. Within this, group dancing facilitated collective social bonding whilst individual dancing was a form of physical performance, self-expression and individuality. Brake notes the importance of the ability to create dance in black communities:

> The ghetto offers a supportive culture which makes a dent in hegemony. Black popular culture, music, dance and style articulates this specifically for youth, creating a 'space' which enables them to resist. ... Dance has taken on primary significance; ... it replaced fighting as a male contest. (1985, p. 126)

The gendered nature of the dance hall and dance as a form of social behaviour within it has been noted by Mungham (1976), Brake (1985), Sherlock (1993) and Kohn (1997), whilst distinctive dance styles were also diffentiated for specific subcultural groups such as punks, mods, rockers, and hip hop break dancers (Brake, 1985). Sociological studies of the body reveal the gendered ways in which women and men are located in the social landscape and their differential occupation of urban space and personal space (Scott and Morgan, 1993). Thus dancing, the experience of individual clubbers and the leisure space they occupy are all tempered by issues such as differential rights of access and 'choice' for women and men in clubland. Women's and men's different spatial presence is illustrated in studies, for example, on men-only clubs (Rogers, 1988), factories (Westwood, 1984), live gigs (Hanna, 1999), American bars (Spradley and Mann, 1975) and British pubs (Hey, 1986; Hunt and Satterlee, 1987; Measham, 1988). The issues of space, safety, and clubbing in the city will be discussed further in Chapter 6.

The rave and dance club scene was notable in its departure from these previous social dance norms and the related gender interaction. For the first time in post-war British dancing, attendance at dance halls and night clubs was not directly related to finding a romantic, sexual or dance partner for significant numbers of young adults of both sexes. Broadly speaking, dancing for oneself rather than the pursuit of partners was the distinctive feature of attendance at raves and dance events from the late 1980s and this was emphasised by both researchers and participants (Henderson, 1993b). Behaviours and attitudes had changed and the differently gendered ambience this created in dance clubs led to relief from obligations, expectations and sexual pressures for both women and men:

> The communal atmosphere of the rave seemed to erode the predatory sexual relations of traditional night-club life and for many women the rave scene opened up access to the kind of thrills and pleasures that had previously been the preserve of masculine subcultures. (Osgerby, 1998, p. 56)

Henderson agrees with Osgerby that the dance club scene offered the possibility of women experiencing new pleasures, pleasures more usually restricted to men's involvement in post-war British youth cultures:

> ... in contrast to other nocturnal leisure pursuits, pride of place is not given to pursuit of a sexual partner in the repertoire of pleasures on offer. ... sensations of the 'Mind, Body or Soul' are the more likely motivation for participating. (Henderson, 1993b, p. 48)

The dance club scene took the notion of individual, unpartnered social dancing one step further than previous youth cultures. Women danced primarily for their own pleasure rather than as a gendered mating performance or visual spectacle. And men danced for pleasure too rather than as partners or spectators to women's dancing.[6] Hanna's notion of the transformative potential of theatrical dance in terms of gender relations and gender norms has some relevance to social dance in 1990s Britain. In the dance club scene, energetic, prolonged, repetitive dancing combined with music, lights, dry ice and the general environment to produce conditions favourable to 'losing oneself' in the dance. Thus dancing facilitated the displacement of self within the dance club and the dislocation of identity, including gender identity. This notion of 'losing oneself' is linked by Stanley to speed and movement, when describing the 'raver' as surrendering to

> the ritual of the undanceable dance in a Dionysian abandonment to a beat that is both unselfconscious and oblivious ... Speed and movement ensure that the self is no longer ... subject to an external gaze, and that there is only the giddy neutralization of self-space in a dissolution of boundaries between public and private, order and disorder. (Stanley, 1997, p. 52)

Henderson echoes Hanna's view of the role of dance in enhancing the fluidity of gender identities:

> ... femininity (and masculinity) in the context of the rave involves a more fragmented set of identities and positions with the potential for more *equal* difference between the sexes. (Henderson, 1993c, p. 125)

This 'gender blurring' on the dance floor led to the regendering of the club dancer as both male and female. Greater participation in dancing by clubbers of all levels of competency as well as both sexes led to an emphasis on participation rather than performance:

... there was a fracturing of the conventions which have commonly structured the body in dance in pop history. Instead of, as usual, the female body being subjected to the ever-present 'look', the dancers ... turned in on themselves ... dancing no longer solely represented the erotic display of the body. (Redhead, 1990, p. 6)

Thus the links between dancing, gender identity and physical pleasure found new forms in dance club culture for both women and men. Some commentators have gone so far as to suggest that the 'gaze' turned inwards and led to a degree of 'auto-eroticism' (Henderson, 1993a, p. 50). Indeed, Reynolds and Press take the notion of auto-eroticism one step further with their radical analysis of male clubbers' discovery of the pleasures of dance, by suggesting rave culture was

clitoris-envy. ... Gay eroticism has filtered, via house and techno, into the body-consciousness of straight, working-class boys, and finds a perfect fit with their homosocial laddishness. Rave culture ... is remarkable for its asexuality; dancers frug and twirl for the self-pleasuring, narcissistic bliss of it, not to attract a potential mate. This 'androgyny' may really be a subconscious attempt to usurp female potencies and pleasures, in order to dispense with real women altogether. (Reynolds and Press, 1995, p. 64)

And the final element in the regendered, increased participation in dance was the added attraction that dancing was exercise. It was a fun form of physical exertion (and almost effortless after consuming dance drugs) and yet it could lead to a degree of physical fitness and even weight loss given the energetic and prolonged nature of this form of dancing in hot and humid conditions. The effects of dancing were further enhanced by the consumption of stimulant dance drugs which increased metabolic rates whilst suppressing appetite. (Gender and dance drug use will be discussed in more detail in the next section.) As Henderson has noted, fun, fitness and weight control made rave dancing particularly attractive to women (Henderson, 1993b). Although to a lesser extent, the fitness element of rave dancing appealed to men too; the slim and toned body of regular male clubbers (predisposed to dancing 'topless' at many 1990s hardcore dance events) was in contrast to the distinctive 'beer bellies' of male drinkers of whom ravers were particularly critical. Early 1990s dance club fashions changed from 'baggy' and bright Mediterranean and hippy-inspired casual wear to sleek and slimfitting sports and club wear. Alongside this, research into the early 1990s dance drug casualties and fatalities implicated overheating and dehydration (Henry, 1992). This resulted in harm reduction advice for dance drug users specifically on what to wear at dance events. Clubbers were encouraged to wear minimal, loose, cool clothing. Thus for both fashion and safety reasons, more of the male and female body was on display on the dance floor by the mid-1990s than in the earlier acid house and rave scenes. Whilst not suggesting that men are equally exposed to social pressures surrounding body image as women in our society, there is evidence that male clubbers had a degree of self-consciousness about their bodies. For example, some young male clubbers used steroids specifically to improve the appearance of their bodies, knowing they would be on display in clubland. In Chapter 5 we will consider the results from the medical component of our study and explore the relationship between dancing, dance drug use and weight loss.

Therefore social dancing at rave/dance events involved both women and men dancing for themselves, in ways unprecedented in post-war British night clubs. Furthermore, there was a transformative potential in the gender blurring which occurred on the dance floor and in gender interactions in dance clubs. But was this differently gendered ambience of clubland temporary and drug-induced, or was it a reflection of wider changes in gender norms in pre-millennial Britain? We will now consider the influence of the consumption of dance drugs on gender interactions and gendered behaviour in dance clubs, and consider further the context and climate of such gender changes in relation to changes in wider society.

Dance drugs

Debate about gender, night clubs and drugs is nothing new. Historically, a recurring twentieth-century concern of the media, politicians and the general public about women dancing at night clubs has been the relative social freedom that occurs, with the potential for different races, genders and socio-economic classes to mix in clubs, with the dynamic added ingredient of intoxication with alcohol or illicit drugs (Kohn, 1992). Such twentieth-century concerns about women and leisure have their origins in nineteenth-century debates about women's presence in public houses, gin palaces and music halls, and wider debates about the perceived immorality and irresponsibility of certain sections of the working classes (Stedman Jones, 1971; Stedman Jones, 1983; Hey, 1986; Measham, 2000). Concerns about young women's attendance at night clubs has linked these leisure locations with increased vulnerability and threats to women's safety, either inside clubs or travelling to and from them. These concerns, particularly on the part of the media, were also evident in the late 1980s and early 1990s in response to women's visibility, and also women's visible drugs consumption, in the dance club scene.

The noticeable participation of women in the dance club scene from the early days of acid house resulted in classic tabloid stories of innocent female victims of male drug dealers, and of female clubbers incapacitated and oblivious to predatory sexual advances as a result of their drug-induced state (Redhead, 1993; Henderson, 1997). Such portrayals of 1980s/90s 'ravers' echoed portrayals of

1920s 'flappers' and the recurrent polarisation of female drug users as either innocent victims lured into the world of drugs by male acquaintances, or as strange, deviant, and 'unfeminine' women by definition because they 'chose' to take drugs and were *not* lured into it. Indeed it has been suggested that Leah Betts, who died after taking ecstasy in 1995, served as an icon of the anti-drugs lobby in much the same way as Freda Kempton, who died after taking cocaine in 1922 (Kohn, 1997). Both deaths were linked to stimulant use, night clubs and birthday parties; both women had knowingly consumed stimulants on previous occasions; and yet both were portrayed as young female 'victims', with their deaths later used by the media and anti-drugs lobby to warn against drugs. The details surrounding both these female drug users' deaths prove more interesting than the 'victim' stereotypes. Although the dancing, recreational stimulant drug use and leisure of both young women were linked with night clubs and both had been out to clubs on the night they fell ill, in fact the last fatal consumption of stimulants for both of them occurred *in their homes*. For Freda Kempton, her consumption of cocaine in her lodgings led to the inquest deciding she had committed suicide (Kohn, 1997). For Leah Betts, her consumption of ecstasy and then excessive water (to counteract nausea resulting from the ecstasy) at her parents' house led to the inquest deciding that she died from water intoxication or hyponatraemia (Maxwell et al., 1993; Collin and Godfrey, 1997; Henry et al., 1998).

For other female drug users, however, those considered to be the bad girls in the 'good girl–bad girl' dichotomy, their pleasure seeking was pathologised and the female raver was linked to the late 1960s term 'raver' which implied sexual availability or excess (Henderson, 1993c). Thus the good girl–bad girl stereotypes applied by the popular press in their analyses of dance club culture explicitly connected women's drug use with women's sexuality (Redhead, 1993; Henderson, 1993c).

There is no doubt that the differently gendered ambience of dance events from the late 1980s was in part a product of the consumption of psycho-active substances by large numbers of people on the dance floor. Two of the most popular illegal dance drugs of the 1990s, ecstasy and amphetamines, were attributed with directly reducing sexual interaction between women and men because of their physiological effects on men, either inhibiting erection or orgasm.[7] Consequently dance club culture has been considered by Reynolds to be the first youth culture where sex was *not* used as a token of symbolic subcultural defiance (Reynolds, 1997). Henderson agrees:

... all this sensuality and hedonism ... was not tied into a straightforward sexual narrative: 'doing' sex had lost its pride of place in the new chemical Britain after dark. (Henderson, 1999, p. 40)

However, whilst a dance club full of customers who predominantly consumed ecstasy and amphetamines undoubtedly felt qualitatively different from a club full of customers who drank alcohol, this was not the result of a simple causal relationship between drugs and sex. Taking a point made by Henderson one step further (1993b), when considering the effects of dance drugs on sexual behaviour we have to consider the complex relationship between pharmacology of individual street drugs of varying quality and composition, preconceptions of psycho-active drugs, actual physiological effects, poly drug use, the drug setting and individual user's mind set, the individual, social and cultural context of both drugs and sexuality, and the interpretation and response of individuals to this combination of drug effects, set, setting, prior learning, and social conditioning. Thus it is problematic to disentangle the social, sexual, sensual and pharmacological factors that make up the whole drugs experience for each person. Indeed, scientific research attempting to assess subjective experiences of drugs intoxication is in its infancy (Stevens, 1987; Newcombe and Johnson, 1999). The lack of social scientific research on subjective drugs experiences and intoxication contrasts with the abundance of writing on subjective drugs experiences in the realms of literature. (For a discussion of fiction, prose and poetry on drugs see, for example, Plant, 1999.)

Reynolds has pointed out how the nature of rave music complemented the anti-aphrodisiac effects of ecstasy and amphetamines so the music and drugs together created a different social space for both female and male clubbers. In this space platonic, physical and sensual contact, rather than sexual interaction, predominated. Thus Reynolds, like Henderson, contends that the traditional sexual narrative of music and clubbing was abolished with dance music

> in favour of an infinitely sustained pre-orgasmic plateau, during which the adept enters a mystic hallucinatory state. Both ecstasy and amphetamine tend to have an anti-aphrodisiac effect. E may be the 'love drug', but this refers more to ... cuddles rather than copulation ... turning rave into space where girls can feel free to be friendly with strange men, even snog them, without fear of sexual consequences. (Reynolds, 1997, p. 106)

As discussed above, this resulted in some women finding dance events preferable to traditional straight night clubs because of the resulting reduction in sexual advances, propositions and harassment from heterosexual men. Gone too were the pressures of sexual initiation and performance for men. Alongside this, female clubbers criticised the traditional sexual narrative in night clubs where alcohol rather than dance drugs played a key role. There was specific criticism of 'beer monsters' with their tell-tale 'beer bellies' who appeared in stark contrast to the lean and toned male clubbers of the 1990s. Henderson's research with clubbers, conducted in 1992, suggested that one appeal of dance clubs was the lack of harassment and the opportunity to meet and make friends with clubbers of both sexes. Henderson's interviews with clubbers involved in the dance club scene revealed the range of sensual experiences on offer, the socialising, and the sense of togetherness with both friends and strangers in clubs which all rated as bigger attractions than meeting sexual partners. Instead, the sensuous and communal rather than sexual attributes of dance drugs, enhanced by the dance music of the time, led to descriptions of asexual tactile interactions between clubbers reminiscent of early adolescence.[8] Physical affection blossomed in clubland without expectations/obligations of escalation, unwanted sexual attention, or the attendant risks of pregnancy, sexually transmitted diseases, HIV/AIDS, or sexual assault. Henderson reported that her own study 'suggests that the "dance drug" phenomenon ... is less likely to provoke unsafe sex than the use of alcohol in large social settings' (1993a, p. 126). Thus a notable distinction of dance clubs was their relative physical safety for women, and also for men too, without the threat of alcohol-related aggression so prevalent in drinking venues (Gofton, 1990; Marsh and Fox Kibby, 1992). This break with traditional night club behaviour by males is illustrated by one male clubber, Russell David:

No one wanted a battle. No one was pissed and falling all over you. All anyone wanted to do was dance. ... I had my hands in the air ... and someone grabbed one of them. ... it was some lad I'd never seen before, and then his mate grabbed my other hand, all of us with our shirts off, hug, and I swear, I wasn't the only one with tears in my eyes. (Quoted in Harrison, 1998, p. 2. Also see Anthony, 1998, pp. 5–9.)

Henderson emphasises the combination of safety and fun in dance clubs:

... the young women occupied this social space with confidence, circulating and meeting new people independently. ... [clubs] provided an exciting, exhilarating but also 'safe' social space for them ... (Henderson, 1993a, p. 125)

Thus dance clubs held a similar appeal for women to gay clubs which have been populated by a minority of heterosexual women alongside lesbians and gay men for years. Gay clubs and dance events can offer straight, lesbian and bisexual women this combination of safety and fun:

... a night of dancing and fun in an environment which does not hold a predictable and oppressive sexual narrative. (Henderson, 1993c, p. 126)

A new physicality and sensuality developed which pointed to a more complex relationship between the physical and psychological effects of psycho-active drugs and male and female sexuality. It was not simply that ecstasy decreased sexual desire in men and therefore men were dancing rather than 'copping off', drinking and fighting. It was not simply that erection, penetration and orgasm-oriented sex was replaced with non-penetrative sex or displaced from Saturday night to Sunday morning. Men did not have to have penetrative sex to prove themselves; women did not have to avoid initiating physical relationships on any level with men for fear of male disapproval or for fear of male expectations on them to have full penetrative sex. There was a new ambience in the gendered social space of clubland, with a lack of obligation or expectation on both sides of the 'gender divide'. In short, men did not need to appear 'ready and willing', and women did not need to fear appearing 'ready and willing'. The implications of this, for a short time, were far-reaching and challenged some of the prevalent masculine and feminine stereotypes of young adult heterosexuality. In this analysis, dance drug use is seen as resulting in disinhibition, tolerance and experimentation in dance club culture leading to the breaking down of some of the more rigid gender norms of behaviour on the dance floor, and also on the football terraces and in the bedroom.

There is a danger of overstating the case here, however. Young people attending dance clubs in the 1990s were not asexual, automaton dance machines. If dance clubs were high on sexual or sensuous feelings but low on sexual activities, there was still the prospect of sexual activity occurring in the 'come down' period, at least for some. Interviews with young clubbers reveal that sex still occurred in the chill out/come down period after clubbing and given the stimulant, empathogenic[9] and hallucinogenic drugs consumed, could become a prolonged, more varied and more significant act than the brief drunken sexual encounters characterised in traditional Saturday night scenarios (Saunders, 1995; Klee, 1998). One example that dance drug users were not asexual dance machines is provided by a question incorporated in Henderson's study of sexuality and recreational drug use in north-west England. Henderson asked 64 young female ecstasy users and 34 young male ecstasy users whether ecstasy made them feel 'horny' never, occasionally, most or all of the time they took it. Given the anti-aphrodisiac perspective discussed above, it is interesting to note that 67 per cent of women and 71 per cent of men reported that they felt 'horny' after taking ecstasy at least occasionally. A quarter of male and female respondents said it varied depending on the brand of ecstasy tablet and dosage. Only 8 per cent of women and 3 per cent of men said they never felt 'horny' after taking ecstasy. Young women at the time were quoted as saying they preferred sex with their male partners on ecstasy because they became more prolonged, sensitive and generous lovers, prioritising their partner's sexual pleasure above their own (Henderson, 1997; Harrison, 1998). Henderson also noted that delayed orgasm or partial erection as a result of dance drug consumption led to greater sexual experimentation with non-penetrative (and therefore safer) sexual practices (1993b).

Changes in social interaction, however, went further than a preponderance for hugging, kissing and massage. Researchers and commentators noted that socialising at clubs was far more fluid than at traditional night clubs and involved mixed sex groups, single sex groups and individuals, rather than couples. Individuals circulated around the dance club socialising with friends and strangers, rather than being tied to one group of friends or one corner of the club. In this way female clubbers accessed social space in new ways in dance clubs. They perceived less social and physical restrictions on their behaviour, they utilised both wider social networks and a greater physical space than at traditional night clubs or pubs (Measham, 1988; Measham, 2000). Indeed such were the changes to gendered interaction within clubland that Henderson went so far as to liken it to a

> feminist dream. It looked like Ecstasy and house culture had provided the landscape, or catalyst even, for social change ... the white flag seemed to be flying in the sex war ... Exploring your sexuality, identity, personal power; pleasuring yourself (and others); being social on a grand stage; having male (body) 'mates' had never been quite like this before for girls. (1997, p. 73)

There were also important gender changes under way for heterosexual men on the dance floor too, as Gilman (1994), Welsh (1995), Saunders (1997), Reynolds (1998) and Henderson (1997, 1999) have noted. A feature of dance clubs was the physical and verbal affection which occurred between heterosexual men (Anthony, 1998). Drawing on the links between gay clubland and rave culture (discussed in more detail later in this chapter), this was notably the only time in the post-war history of British social dance that hugging, kissing and massage, with both friends and strangers, with both the same sex and opposite sex, was possible without heterosexual men's sexuality being called into question. During the honeymoon period of ecstasy culture, when even football 'hooligans' were luv'd up on the dance floor, this atmosphere carried through to their behaviour outside clubs, at least in the short term. (Indeed, ecstasy and dance culture have been attributed as contributory factors in the decline of football hooliganism in Britian in the mid-1990s (Gilman, 1994; Henderson, 1997).) The dilution of ecstasy culture, however, has not been linked to the rise in alcohol-related violence by young people in recent crime figures.) In part these changes in men's behaviour and attitude were seen as a direct consequence of the consumption of ecstasy (Anthony, 1998). But what was the significance of the wider changes affecting men at this time? Henderson believes that this 'makeover ... [of] modern manhood' (1997, p. 95) was more than simply the 'luv'd up' pharmacological effects of ecstasy; it also related to changing perceptions of masculinity and its relationship to broader socio-economic changes in the 1990s.

The wider context for the differently gendered ambience of 1990s dance clubs was one in which men and masculinities were undergoing change (Segal, 1990; Campbell, 1993; Connell, 1993; Marsiglio, 1995; Walby, 1999). For example, the changing socio-economic climate brought changing education and employment opportunities for women and men. Increased male unemployment, alongside the erosion of the concepts, if never the reality, of the male breadwinner and the job-for-life occurred in tandem with increased female (principally part-time, low paid) employment so that women make up over half of the labour force at the start of the twenty-first century (Williams, 1993; Füredi, 1995). Equal opportunities were increasingly related to men's and fathers' rights alongside women's and mothers' rights (Bertoia and Drakich, 1995). Shared parenting, portfolio careers, short-term contracts, maternity and paternity leave, and more women than men in the labour force all hinted at changes in the climate of gender relations in employment, if not in the domestic arena. The 'new man', although initially an advertising construct and media label, exemplified a new permission for (some) men to be emotionally expressive (see Carrigan et al., 1985). It was against this backdrop that the 'nocturnal genderscape' changed (Henderson, 1997, p. 96). We will now discuss some of the issues surrounding the 'nocturnal genderscape' of British clubland in relation to gender, different sub-genres of dance music and the consumption of dance drugs.

Music commentators on dance club culture have (somewhat mechanistically) linked dance drugs, dance music and the gendered attitudes and behaviour of clubbers across the 'decade of dance'. Thus the first two waves of rave were characterised by the 'luv'd up' ecstasy culture, which was then seen as splitting into two branches, mellow house and hardcore, in the early 1990s. This split involved the development of two distinctive tempos, with the 'beats per minute' of dance music spanning from about 120 beats per minute with house music, up to 160 beats per minute or more with hardcore. Commentators have identified a pharmaceutical shift corresponding with the development of the hardcore/mellow split in dance music, with speed replacing what were perceived to be increasingly dubious quality and content ecstasy tablets as the central dance drug. Larger quantities of amphetamines were being consumed on the hardcore scene, and also growing use of cocaine and to a lesser extent crack (Headon, 1994; Saunders, 1995; James, 1997). This resulted in what has been described as a new speed-freak hardcore subculture (Reynolds and Press, 1995). More moderate dance drug use,[10] a return to alcohol and an increase in cocaine use were seen as the key pharmaceutical distinctions of the mellow dance club scene. The 'luv'd up' ecstasy vibe was retreating from the dance scene and alongside it the collective social bonding between women and men which had been a distinctive feature of the earlier dance club culture. Replacing the luv'd up vibe, according to Reynolds and Press, was sexless disconnection:

Amphetamine promotes sexless concentration, single-minded focus; ... Suffice it to say that if disconnection 'is the genius of patriarchy', as Robin Morgan claims, then speed is the ultimate patriarchal drug. (Reynolds and Press, 1995, p. 63)

Henderson noted that whilst she wanted to avoid being too deterministic in the influence of different dance music types on gendered behaviour in dance clubs, nevertheless there was a divide betweeen mellow and hardcore, between what she called softer house or garage and the harsher sounds of techno. It was at the so-called techno clubs that men could be found dancing all night on dance drugs. Thus she concluded it was possible to identify some distinctions in drug use and related behaviour in different sub-genres of dance club. More recently, O'Hagan has maintained the techno–garage distinction in dance music in his study of late 1990s British dance culture and associated drug use in eight London clubs. He found differences between clubbers attending the two different types of dance club in both lifetime prevalence of drug use and in drugs taken or planned for the fieldwork night (O'Hagan, 1999). Those customers attending techno clubs reported more widespread use of a wider range of illicit drugs than at the garage clubs, with higher rates of self-reported consumption/planned consumption of cannabis, ecstasy, amphetamine, LSD and ketamine on the fieldwork night. Customers at garage clubs had higher self-reported levels of alcohol and cocaine use/planned use on the fieldwork night.

Garratt takes Reynolds and Press' gender analysis of the sexless speed-freak hardcore scene one step further. She suggests that men's drug-induced lack of interest in female clubbers combined with the alienating nature of aggressive hardcore dance music and resulted in lower women's attendance at hardcore dance events as the 'decade of dance' wore on:

... the various strands of this collapsing rave scene developed into genres of their own. ... Most of these scenes became overwhelmingly male, as women began to find them increasingly unappealing: rendered temporarily incapable of sex by their chemical intake, few of the lads sweating it out on the dancefloor actually seemed to notice they'd gone. (Garratt, 1998, p. 271)

This is a somewhat ahistoric, pharmaceutically determined analysis of the cultural shifts in the dance club scene. If we consider the development of hardcore dance music and specifically 'dark side' or 'dark core', with its use of horror and science fiction imagery, it has been seen as representing the unease of this period and dramatising a fragmenting social scene. Fisher, for example, sees dark side as giving a voice to the 'dread' of 1990s Britain, to the rapid socio-economic change taking place, the corresponding changes in men's lives in particular, and the resulting sense of uncertainty about the future. Perhaps easy to minimise with hindsight, the following quote captures the sense of turmoil of the mid-1990s:

> In 1994, change is everywhere, at such a rate that few can yet assimilate what's happening. Institutions that seemed solid – the royal family, the family itself – are crumbling. The postulations of postmodernist theory about the decline of grand narratives, of feminist theory about the redundancy of the male, are becoming lived social reality. ... Dark Side's dread futurism invites us to recognise the way things are mutating. Our horror might only be the death throes of the old order. (Fisher, 1994, p. 33)

What is interesting is the possibility that this particular sub-genre of hardcore dance music – dark side – developed within the context of, and reflected, wider social change at this time, including changes in gender norms and gender relations. In this analysis the differently gendered ambience of 1990s hardcore dance clubs reflects changes in wider society rather than being solely the product of psycho-active drug use and the distinctions of a particular youth culture. This challenges the perspective of commentators such as Garratt above, which portrays hardcore as a simple reassertion of working-class masculinity and the end of the communal luv'd up atmosphere because of a reduction in ecstasy consumption. For other commentators and particularly for those male and female clubbers who attended hardcore dance events, hardcore was seen as a continuation of the rave ethos rather than overthrowing it. Rather than a reassertion of gender identity and the polarised constraints of masculinity and femininity, Reynolds and Press suggest that hardcore *epitomised* the notion of 'losing oneself' in the music – an element of dance club culture since its inception – an implosion of the self even to the extent of losing one's gender identity, one's sexuality, and one's sensuality:

> ... the rise of 'ardkore was perceived as a swing towards a more masculine aesthetic (harder, faster, noisier, brutal, anti-melodic). For some it was a degeneration from the polymorphous sensuality of earlier rave music, ... But the sublimity of pure speed is as much a longing for ego dissolution as a hypermasculine assertion of self. The urge to surge and the urge to merge fuse in a raging oceanic feeling. In 'ardkore's chaotic swirl, you become an androgyne. (Reynolds and Press, 1995, p. 64)

Sometimes lost in the analysis of hardcore dance and dance drugs is the fact that women also attended hardcore dance events and also consumed these dance drugs. Although variations in quantity, frequency and types of dance drugs consumed by women existed, empirical studies suggest that there was no general decline in women's drug use throughout the 1990s (Parker et al., 1998; Ramsay and Partridge, 1999). This had an impact not just on the dance floor but also in the field of gender and drugs research. Research on gender and drugs in the 1980s consisted mostly of critiques of the previous 'mad, sad or bad' research on women and drugs. The stereotypes of the 'mad, sad or bad' women drug users tap into the deeply embedded religious and philosophical perspectives of Christian societies since the Middle Ages that the recreational use of psycho-active drugs, and indeed all bodily pleasures and the resulting loss of self-control, can be morally questionable (Foucault, 1976, 1984). The intensities of passion and delirium were seen as the basis and prerequisite for irrationality, irresponsibility, immorality and ultimately madness in the Age of Reason (Foucault, 1961).[11] In this analysis the active pursuit of physical pleasure in Western societies is considered to be deviant, weak or immoral.

Research in the 1990s attempted to re-introduce notions of agency into women's drug use (Taylor, 1993; Maher, 1997; Henderson, 1993a, 1993b, 1993c, 1997; Parker et al., 1998). Influenced by research within the field of cultural studies, notions of consumption and pleasure rather than dependency and problematic drug use are now being considered in relation to women's drug use. The contrast between the two notions of pleasurable and problematic female drug use is most noticeable with female dance drug users, who cannot be categorised as either caricature of problematic female drug users: pathologically deranged addicts or innocent victims of male dealers. In her seminal work on young women's recreational drug use and sexuality in the rave scene, Henderson explicitly put Ettore's plea into practice for more discussion of the pleasures of women's drug use (Ettore, 1992). When Henderson discussed the features of dance culture, which included dancing, music, drug use, social interaction, physical affection, auto-eroticism, and flirtation, she located pleasure at its centre (1997). Henderson portrayed female dance drug users as active consumers in pursuit of pleasure for themselves, rather than the more usual stereotypes of women giving or receiving pleasure. However, in following Ettore and emphasising the pleasure-seeking motivations of her female clubbers, Henderson runs the risk of feeding the negative stereotype of the selfishly pleasure-seeking female drug user, even if Henderson's intention was to portray a positive feminist slant to their pleasure seeking.

In her most recent work Henderson has called for a consideration of issues of drugs and gender which reaches beyond women's drug use as the subject of study. She suggests instead the exploration of subjects such as broader social trends, changes in femininity *and* masculinity and their links to the gendered use of drugs in millennial Britain (Henderson, 1999). Looking back on the female clubbers she interviewed in the early 1990s who went out and enjoyed themselves, took drugs and danced all night, Henderson sees these young women as cultural consumers rather than drug addicts and perhaps even as fore-runners of late 1990s 'girl power' (a term popularised by the British five-piece 'girl band' called the Spice Girls in the late 1990s). The shift from drug users as 'addicts' to 'consumers' is conceptually important but not the full story, however. The behaviour of these early 1990s clubbers can now be more clearly linked to socio-economic changes for women, as we have considered above for men in the hardcore scene. The increase in education and employment opportunities for some women led to higher expectations for many more. Yet women's earnings remain about three-quarters of men's in millennial Britain, with the perpetuation of occupational sex segregation and women clustered at lower levels of income prompting renewed efforts by the most recent Labour government to address gender inequalities (EOC, 1999). The differential impact of socio-economic changes on different sections of society means choice, including choice in relation to drug use, is not equally shared by all those within and on the margins of consumer society (Cahill, 1994; Gibbins and Reimer, 1999). The changing nature of women's, as well as men's, drug use must be located within the context of broader socio-economic changes in the 1990s and needs to be understood as such, not simply as a lifestyle choice.

And what of gender and dance club culture at the turn of the century? Henderson, Garratt and other commentators have noted that with the popularisation, commercialisation and fragmentation of the dance scene, there was also an increasing sexualisation. The late 1990s have been characterised by the re-emergence of the traditional heterosexual narrative, with the atmosphere in clubland shifting from 'luv'd up' to 'sex'd up' (Henderson, 1997). Henderson points out that elements of the re-emergence of sex were evident in club clothes, professional dancers and club flyers from as early as 1993 (1993b). Where once women's skimpy club clothes were functional and liberating, the tone became more sexist and exploitative, as was evident in promotional materials, posters, flyers and advertisements for clubs. It was also apparent in the discussions between clubbers and club promoters published in the letters pages of dance music magazines such as *Muzik* (April, 1996; June, 1996). Previously innovative club nights such as Manumission became known for nightly live sex shows on stage in Ibiza. Again there was a pharmaceutical determinism in interpretations of changing club culture, with the changing gendered ambience in clubland being seen as the direct result of shifting patterns of dance drug use:

> This sexiness is probably a side-effect of British clubbers' shift of allegiance from anti-aphrodisiac Ecstasy to horny-making cocaine. (Reynolds, 1998, p. 420)

As dance clubs in the late 1990s became more mainstream, commercial and conventional their early optimism and transformative potential seemed to be replaced, but was it by a new sexist realism or a return to the nocturnal genderscape of old? The switch from grassroots male and female clubbers up to corporate music industry males has led to the re-gendering of the dance floor and some might claim a return to traditionally gendered pre-1990s club culture. With clubbers no longer the stars on the dance floors, without the short-lived luv'd up ecstasy culture and the ripples of the rave ethos, clubbers became consumers of club culture, spectators rather than participants. As Garratt notes of house clubs after 1995:

> These were not places for clubbers to experiment, to try out new sexual and cultural identities. ... Less participants *creating* the spectacle, more consumers now expecting to have it created for them ... (Garratt, 1998, p. 303)

Commercialisation overshadowed democratisation on the dance floor. Such consumerism and excess in late pre-millennial clubland has been compared to the 'last days of disco' and has led to much criticism of the 'superclubs' (Naylor, 1996; Benson, 1996; Garratt, 1998).

So 1990s dance culture and the differently gendered social space of dance clubs may have been only a temporary break with previous youth cultures but Henderson does not see this as a short-lived fluke for women or for men. Henderson sees these gendered changes in club culture as part of a broader picture of socio-economic change, and symptomatic of broader changes in gender relations towards the millennium.

Given the increasingly multifaceted nature of millennial dance club culture, however, it is difficult to generalise about gender in clubland. What is interesting is that whilst media and public concerns around gender, drugs and clubs focus on women's vulnerability, one of the distinctive features of gender interaction within the rave/dance club scene has been safety, with a reduced fear of sexual assault for women and reduced fear of violent assault for men. For the first time, clubs were safe *and* fun, for women *and* men. New horizons of experimentation rather than expectation facilitated a fluidity in social interactions and gender relations which developed through sensuous, 'safer', asexual, androgynous or auto-erotic forms of expression. This newly gendered dance club culture was centred on pleasure: the rediscovery of physical, sensuous pleasure for women and men which was produced by both dancing and dance drugs, and the entwining of the two. (Perceptions of safety in clubland is a theme we will return to when we look at the views of the respondents in this research study in Chapter 6.)

Having considered gender in clubland, we now go on to consider socio-economic class where again the early transformative potential of club culture was dispersed in later years.

Socio-economic class: revenge of the suburbs

Debates about the relationship between youth culture and socio-economic class can be traced back to the 1970s sociology of deviance, with studies of most previous youth cultures suggesting they were predominantly working class. (For 1970s theoretical discussion of the complexities of the relationship between class and youth cultures see for example Cohen, 1972; Clarke et al., 1976; Murdock and McCron, 1976; Clarke and Jefferson, 1976.) Well-worn paths trace the development of these working-class youth cultures and their links to the dislocation of traditional working-class communities and growing post-war affluence, alongside parallel developments in mass manufacturing and marketing. Higher levels of routine, boredom and exploitation at work led to increasing preoccupation with, and possibilities for, weekend leisure and lifestyles. As such, working-class youth cultures were seen both as symbols of post-war social change in Britain, and also as sites for cultural class conflict (Cohen, 1971; Clarke and Critcher, 1985). The possible class exceptions to this were the predominantly middle-class student protest movements, bohemian lifestyles and counter-cultures of the middle-class intelligentsia such as the hippies of the late 1960s and early 1970s (Brake, 1985). Although there were suggestions about the 'classless', consumerist nature of youth culture with the development of the consumer category of 'teenager', challenges to this notion and the reassertion of the predominantly working-class core of British youth cultures are a theme of studies from the Centre for Contemporary Cultural Studies onwards (Clarke and Jefferson, 1976; Hebdige, 1979; Brake, 1985). Indeed, the implication is that the experience of being working class in itself was central to the formation of British youth cultures. 'Youth ... are responding to the specific contradictory features of the world of working class youth' (Clarke and Jefferson, 1976, p. 151).

The early rave/dance culture has been seen as a continuation of that vibrant post-war tradition of working-class culture and collective organisation. Within the rave scene the threads of working-class youth culture were identified:

> Like football fandom, rave is a remnant of working-class consciousness, the vague sense of collectivity that abides after the death of organized labour with all its myths of fraternity and shared destiny. (Reynolds, 1997, p. 110)

Other commentators have suggested that the early rave scene was a distinctive break from preceding youth cultures precisely because it was without the distinct socio-economic base, values and outlook of previous cultural forms. It had neither the boundaries nor the collective conscious identity of a working-class youth culture. It was more diverse, open, inclusive and eclectic than that, and therefore it broke with previous subcultural lineage in its class composition and its class outlook. Newcombe, for example, notes that:

> Though ravers (at least in the North West) are predominantly young working class adults, group membership and shared beliefs are not as important as in

other popular cultures. The hallmark of raves is that people of different ages, occupational groups, sexualities, subcultures and races dance together ... (Newcombe, 1992a, p. 22)

A third perspective is that dance culture was not limited to the street styles of British cities as many previous youth cultures had been. There was a demographic composition to the dance club community which reached beyond the working class and appealed to southern and suburban middle-class youth, unprecedented in the history of youth culture. This was seen as the first youth culture to span all social classes (Kohn, 1997). This is supported in the writings of Garratt and Baker. Looking at the computerised membership list for one particular rave organisation, Sunrise, they noted:

> ... a surprising cross-section of people: bankers and barrow-boys, Sharons and Selinas can all put on the uniform and blend in as long as they have the admission price and the transport to get there. ... The current rave culture is ... the revenge of the suburbs ... In a club culture where mobility is essential, the suburbs rule. (Garratt and Baker, 1989, p. 108)

Thus the broader socio-economic composition of the early rave scene was linked to the mobility of clubbers, who could live anywhere in the country, drive to dance venues and consume illegal drugs with (relatively) little fear of prosecution. This mobility was the result of both the location of dance venues and the consumption of illegal drugs. Firstly, from the early days of raves in disused warehouses, fields and caves, access to transport was important (and continues to be, as we shall see in the distances travelled by respondents to the three clubs in this study). Party venues were revealed on telephone answering machines or pirate radio stations on the very night of the dance event in order to evade police detection, necessitating driving many miles to remote locations (Collin and Godfrey, 1997). Secondly, there was increasingly vigilant policing of drink-driving laws from the late 1980s, without concurrant vigilant policing of drug-driving laws, partly because the scale of driving under the influence of illegal drugs was not yet realised and partly because once it was, the police had no effective roadside drivers' test for suspected drugs consumption in the same way as they had with the breathalyser. Effectively this gave clubbers consuming dance drugs a carte blanche to drive hundreds of miles to dance venues of their choice across the country, a stark comparison with young people consuming alcohol who were restricted to dance venues within walking distance or affordable taxi fare of home. An indication of the significance of the new mobile clubber of the 1990s who was prepared to drive to dance events across the country can be seen in the marketing of illegal drugs: the M25 motorway was such a feature of clubbers' travel that a brand of ecstasy tablet in the early 1990s was called 'M25'. Alongside the car, it has been suggested that ecstasy, too, played a pivotal role in the socio-economic diversity and tolerance of clubbers. Reynolds, for example, considers that any cross-class unity which existed in the early rave scene was a fragile construction which quickly collapsed when the ecstasy consumption stopped and 'rave's E-sponsored unity inevitably refractured along class, race and regional lines' (Reynolds, 1997, p. 103).

Whether or not the early ravers spanned broader socio-economic groupings than previous youth cultures, by the early 1990s the fragmentation into sub-genres of dance music was accompanied by fragmenting social scenes. It was the hardcore branch of dance, rather than the mellow branch, which was perceived to be a working-class collective cultural expression. As discussed in more detail elsewhere in this chapter, the hardcore and particularly the 'darkcore' or dark jungle thread of 1990s dance culture was seen as reflecting the economic pessimism of the black and white working class, or even underclass, of British cities at that time. Again, the customer base of hardcore dance events and of specialist music magazines in the mid-1990s provides evidence of this.

Indeed, such were the links of hardcore dance music with the underclass and its associations with excessive drugs consumption, criminal gangs and related trouble, alongside low alcohol sales and low takings (except for admission fees), that by the mid-1990s some clubs shifted their music policy to more mellow dance sounds such as house and garage. These sub-genres of dance music were perceived to attract more stylish and sophisticated customers than hardcore; customers who it was hoped would take fewer drugs, drink more alcohol, boost profit margins and reduce drug- and gang-related trouble in clubs. The change in music policy was an attempt to change the class base of customers and to draw back the drinking, paying, employed and up-market crowd. In these instances, club music policy was used directly to determine, attract or deter specific customer profiles.

By the late 1990s, the dance club scene had expanded into the pre-eminent and pervasive popular music form of the millennial era. This has been discussed in terms of a new cultural classlessness, the classlessness of fashionable youth, or at least a new consumer dance culture where subcultural capital has overshadowed socio-economic capital (Bourdieu, 1984; Thornton, 1995). Newcombe described the change to consumer culture thus:

Rather than fading away, ... the rave changed its status from a cliquey, mutating underground subculture to a more socially diverse, stable and consumerist popular leisure culture, blurring the boundaries between such previously disparate groups as football fans and various pop music 'tribes'. (Newcombe, 1992a, p. 22)

In such changing times, Thornton questions the relevance of dichotomies used in the study of popular culture in the 1970s and 1980s – such as mainstream/sub-cultural, commercial/alternative and conformity/individualism – to the organisation of dance club culture in 1990s Britain. Whilst recognising that these terms still have relevance for clubbers themselves, Thornton suggests instead the notion of cultural plurality to indicate the complexity and fluidity of current trends. In her exploration of the term 'mainstream', Thornton prob-lematises any simplistic identification of a 'mainstream' crowd in over two hundred clubs which were included in her study:

> To apply the label 'mainstream' to any of these would have run the risk of den-igrating or normalizing the crowd in question. I could always find something that distinguished them – if not local differences, then shades of class, education and occupation, gradations of gender and sexuality, hues of race, ethnicity or religion. (Thornton, 1995, pp. 106–7)

Thus within the broad-based popularity of the spectrum of dance culture, if one looks closely at the distinctions of specific sub-genres and even closer at specific clubs, one may well identify distinctions of class. This is discussed further in relation to one specific example – jungle, race and class – in the next section.

Race: black soundtracks to white leisure

As we shall see throughout this chapter, if key features of the original dance club scene were that it was broadly based in terms of socio-economic class, gender and sexual orientation, the same could not be said for race. That is not to say that black music cultures have not had a presence in dance clubs and dance music – the very opposite. So much dance music played in British clubs throughout this century has derived from African, Caribbean, Asian and black European roots, from jazz to the jitterbug, from soul to swing, that it would be an impossible task to disentangle these influences. Although little has been written about ethnicity and youth culture and even less about ethnicity and dance club culture, there has at least been some recognition of the historical black African and Caribbean contributions. Shapiro, for example, notes the 'long-established tradition whereby British music fans have embraced American black music often far more enthusiastically than the home base' (1999, pp. 20–1). Collin and Godfrey concur:

> Right through ... post-war pop culture, from rock'n'roll, R&B, soul and funk to house and techno, black music has soundtracked white youth's leisure activities and provided the basis for white pop, particularly within dance clubs. (Collin and Godfrey, 1997, p. 259)

When discussing black contributions to dance music, however, there has been some criticism of presumptions that this is taken to mean specifically African and Caribbean contributions. Asian contributions to the British dance scene are notably absent from such discussions (Huq, 1996). It is only the emergence of the new Asian dance music, the so-called 'new Asian Kool' or the 'Asian Underground', that has led to some discussion of such Asian contributions. (Most recently, the growing mainstream recognition of Asian dance music is evident in the 1999 Mercury Music Prize, won by Talvin Singh in September 1999, an artist who combines Asian dance music with British jungle.) New Asian dance music was the product of such diverse influences as Bhangra, Bollywood musicals, and the 1980s Bengali sound systems of East London. The prominence of Asian dance clubs in the early rave scene can be followed from the mixed–gay night Shakti opening in January 1989, continuing with Kali and Anokha, through to the famous weekly Bhangra rave, Bombay Jungle, launched at The Wag in 1993; yet Asian contributions are rarely featured in the 'decade of dance' retrospectives.

Claims for the lineage of rave music back to its black roots might be even clearer than for some other genres within popular music. There are several reasons for this. Firstly, rave music is based on rhythm rather than melody, like certain non-Western, tribal and indigenous music. Secondly, the use of sampling in dance music is seen as grounding itself in black musical–cultural traditions:

> ... revisiting and revising earlier musical work ... a conscious preoccupation with artistic continuity and connection to Black cultural roots. (Smitherman, 1997, pp. 15–16)

Thirdly, dance floor etiquette and forms of crowd response to dance tracks played at clubs, particularly in the hardcore sub-genres of dance such as jungle, happy hardcore and techno, link back to black dance hall traditions: such as the use of MCs (master of ceremonies, or mike chanting), cigarette lighters, DJ rewinds of popular tracks and even on occasion gunshots in the air (for example at the Lighthouse, Manchester, see Newsome, 1996).

Fourthly, the distinctive creative role of the engineer in dance music harks back to the engineer in earlier black musical forms such as reggae. The elevation of technology to a creative force and of the engineer implementing a vision by harnessing that force is an unusually distinctive feature. Furthermore, the very idea of music technology as 'science' has a musical lineage from (black) dub reggae, house and techno to (white) British rave. The use of scientific imagery and terminology in artists, tracks, albums and compilations has now saturated the dance market (see Reynolds, 1999, pp. 202–4 for examples). This leads to the emergence of the engineer as mad scientist, techno-artist or techno-poet:

In today's dance music, the domain of creativity is vested in sound-in-itself ... the realm of the engineer. ... The figure of the engineer-poet first emerged in black music. (Reynolds, 1999, p. 202)

Fifthly, the trademark hardcore dance events' use of MCs who rap or toast over the DJs' music and mixing echoes the use of rap in hip hop. Although the majority of the MCs' audience is white at all but jungle (and more recently UK garage) dance events, the majority of British MCs are black. This results in the language, style and content of the MCs' patter being drawn from black linguistic practices, terminology and lifestyles. Smitherman has identified the black communicative practices in hip hop – many of which can also be identified in black British MCs – which she suggests are methods of rejecting white European linguistic domination. For example, the black oral tradition evident in American rap and British MCs includes tonal semantics, braggadocio, narrativising, signification, the dozens, Africanised syntax, and semantic inversion (Smitherman, 1997). Thus black British hardcore dance MCs, like black Amercian rappers, could be seen as reflecting

the cultural evolution of the Black oral tradition and the construction of a contemporary resistance rhetoric. (Smitherman, 1997, p. 21)

This is supported by James' description of black ragga MCs in British dance halls of the late 1980s, and their 'redeployment of the patois language of resistance' (James, 1997, p. 32).

The history of black music is entwined with the history and experiences of slavery, imperialism, migration and racism (Chambers, 1976). This is eloquently illustrated in McRobbie's description of Jah Wobble's 'dance dub' bass playing where 'the thudding bass line ... told a story of class and history, of manual labour and then later of urban multi-culturalism' (McRobbie, 1999, p. 46). Against this political backdrop, urban leisure spaces such as pubs and clubs provide the public arenas for black cultural forms. It has been suggested that this space in which white and black populations meet, of white racism and black resistance, is

the site of the most acute forms of white racism and syncretic black musical cultures and these continue to thrive both because of, and in spite of, their proximity to each other. (Banerjea and Barn, 1996, p. 198)

Thus the social and political context for a black presence in dance clubs in British cities is a significant part of the creative process itself. Indeed it is a form of racism by white, working-class young men which defines aspects of Afro-Caribbean culture as masculine, militant, sexually potent 'black cool', and yet aspects of Asian culture are seen as alien, effeminate and until the 1990s, definitely 'uncool' (Jones, 1988; Banerjea and Barn, 1996).

There has been a black and ethnic minority presence on British dance floors since the first post-war immigrants came from colonial and post-colonial South Asia and the Caribbean. In the 1960s, for example, Jamaican rude boys were an integral part not only of the black London club scene but also the white mod club scene, and were emulated in clothes, conversation and carriage by white skinheads in the late 1960s (Hebdige, 1976b; Osgerby, 1998). There was also a small black presence in the warehouses, fields and dance floors of the early rave/dance scene (Anthony, 1998), although the size of the black and ethnic minority presence depended in part on locality, music policy and door policy at dance events. However, with a few notable exceptions the first waves of rave were a predominantly white dance culture in terms of both organisation and participation:

> Black men are often barred from city-centre nightspots for spurious reasons; black and white may have danced together at raves, but generally on white terms, with whites in the majority, and whites taking the proceeds. (Collin and Godfrey, 1997, p. 259)

Garratt and Baker also noted that 'the early scene was very white' (1989, p. 108). But if the early rave/dance scene was not genuinely multiracial, things started to change in 1991. Jungle, a 'mainly black form of rave' (James, 1997, p. 3), allowed a significant black presence in rave/dance club culture for the first time.

The term 'jungle' had its roots *geographically* in both the inner city urban jungle/concrete jungle of early 1990s Britain, and in the district of Tivoli Gardens, in Kingston, Jamaica known as the jungle in 'yard' terminology and which was referred to on Jamaican sound system tapes heard back in Britain. *Musically*, references to the concrete or urban jungle can be found in black music as diverse as The Wailers, Sly and the Family Stone and Grandmaster Flash and the Furious Five. *Politically* the term jungle could be seen as a black reappropriation of a previously derogatory word. 'Jungle fever', for example, was a derogatory term for interracial relationships used by Louis Farrakhan of the Nation of Islam and picked up by racists. 'Jungle Jim' was rhyming slang for a 'Tim' or Catholic in mainland Britain. (For a discussion of the origins and political/race implications of the term 'jungle' see James, 1997, and Reynolds, 1998.) The timing of this musical development has been linked to the decline in ecstasy use and its 'luv'd up' vibe, and the implications of this for the young black population of inner-city Britain:

> As hardcore evolved into jungle, it shed rave's emotional demonstrativeness and gestural abandon, which had originated in gay disco and entered white

working-class body-consciousness via Ecstasy. ... the disappearance of the Ecstasy vibe allowed young black Britons to enter the rave scene *en masse* and begin the transformation of hardcore into jungle. Ecstasy's effects of defence-less candour are probably too risky a cultural leap for the young black male, who can't afford to jeopardize the psychic armour necessitated by the very different black experience of urban life. (Reynolds, 1997, pp. 250–1)[12]

Ecstasy and speed were replaced by the new dance drugs of choice in the jungle scene: cannabis, cocaine, alcohol and to a lesser extent, crack. Indeed jungle was blamed in the music press for bringing crack into clubland and ruining the 'happy' vibe in the dance scene. More realistically, changes in both the drugs and the music were themselves part of a broader shift from the euphoric optimism of the early dance scene to a new urban realism, which itself was a reflection of a new realism in wider British society.

The significance of jungle in terms of ethnicity and dance culture has largely gone unnoticed with a few exceptions (Saunders, 1995; Banerjea and Barn, 1996). It was both an exciting, genuinely black British dance music and it was also an indigenous soundtrack for 1990s inner-city Britain (for profiles and photographs of the key DJs, MCs, record producers and label owners, see the 'Who's Who in Jungle' articles in *Generator*, 1995, and *True*, 1996). Jungle drew its appreciation from black and white urban working-class adults, from across a far broader age and ethnicity spectrum than the earlier years of the dance club scene:

Jungle is often hailed as the first significant and truly indigenous Black British music. ... the *multiracial* nature of the scene ... contrasted with the mostly white audience for trance techno and ambient. ... because there's a genuine unity of experience shared by Britain's black and white underclass. (Reynolds, 1997, pp. 247–8)

There were elements of the underclass, the outlaw, in jungle from its inception, as Collin and Godfrey identify:

... a polyrhythmic blend of influences ... a melting pot of urban signals and styles ... jungle was a historic sound: the first truly *British* black music ... Just like hip hop in America, jungle articulated the repressed desires and fears of a disenfranchised underclass. ... Jungle was another example of how black youth subcultures are initially feared and demonised before ultimately being packaged and commercially exploited by the white mainstream. (Collin and Godfrey, 1997, pp. 260–1)

It is interesting to note that whilst some clubbers and commentators viewed jungle as vibrant, radical and the most creative dance sub-genre to emerge from the early waves of rave, many more saw it as aggressive, threatening, savage and 'other': eating away at pure (white) British rave culture (Banerjea and Barn, 1996). Race and drugs combined to form a familiar discourse around the threatening foreign 'invasion'. The debates filled dance music magazines for months. These racialised reactions to the early jungle scene, to the Afro-Caribbean and Asian 'natives' on the dance floors, provide a clear indication of the implicitly white undertones of the earlier rave scene. Jungle

> continues to be stalked by the fears borrowed from an earlier colonial setting. The dislike of jungle translates into fear of the Alien Ruffneck, of the Rudeboy from the council estate who's supposedly spoilt the peace-and-love vibe and the dream of trans-tribal unity. ... It is Jungle that disrupts the ordered progress of British culture. Or so the story goes. (Banerjea and Barn, 1996, p. 214)

An alternative analysis is that the rave scene had become commercialised by the early 1990s and alongside this came compromise, insincerity, fads and fashions with an uncreative alliance of dance drugs and music. In this analysis the hardcore scene, rather than smothering the happy vibe, is seen by some commentators as the genuine descendant of the early rave scene. With hardcore, many of those involved in DJing and production since the early years had 'watched the music mutate from a drug-obsessed mess into something more mature, street-wise and subtle' in jungle (Marcus, 1994).

Therefore, just as the dance scene evolved through women's presence in rave, so the dance scene also evolved through black people's presence in jungle. From its initially predominantly white audience, the dance scene fractured into a multiplicity of sub-genres evident in music, clubs, clothes, and audience profile. Whilst the influences and appropriation of black musical cultures were acknowledged across dance music, it was only in specific dance sub-genres, for example in radical and innovative areas such as jungle and the Asian underground, that black and ethnic minority participation at all levels of dance culture – from production to performance to participation – was evident.

Gay and lesbian clubbing

In contrast to all the previous British youth cultures, with the possible exception of New Romantics, gay men and lesbians had a high profile from the earliest days of the rave/dance club scene. And whilst there have been crossovers between the straight and gay club scenes going back to 1970s discos, glam rock and 'gender bending', British club culture had never been so closely interwoven with the gay scene as during the 'decade of dance'. Retrospectives which discuss the origins of the late 1980s dance music and dance drug scene acknowledge the ways in which it rippled out from a predominantly gay base and indeed note how some of the embryonic features of the dance club scene were evident in gay and lesbian clubs many years earlier. This lineage, from 1970s gay clubs to 1970s discos, 1980s house/garage clubs, late 1980s raves and the current dance scene, will be discussed below.

Pubs and clubs have been a central feature of post-war lesbian and gay culture, a primary meeting place and focus for lesbians and gays in cities across the world. Gay pubs and clubs have the potential to represent a refuge or oasis from a heterosexual/heterosexist world, providing a social space in which to meet friends and partners, dance, and cruise. However, there are several problems inherent in the centrality of gay pubs and clubs to gay leisure. For example, firstly, there is a public health debate about the prevalence of alcohol and drug problems in a community whose central social spaces revolve around licensed premises (see *Journal of Homosexuality*, 1982; *Journal of Chemical Dependency Treatment*, 1992). Secondly, profits go to the corporate drinks and leisure companies, with few managers of gay pubs and clubs being lesbian or gay themselves and few profits being reinvested back into the gay and lesbian communities. (Although there is anecdotal evidence of a growing number of managers and owners of gay pubs and clubs themselves being gay and lesbian.) Thirdly, pubs and clubs are clearly identifiable gay 'targets' leading to discriminatory policing, harassment and 'queer bashing', therefore indicating their symbolic importance as social spaces.[13] In the States Riddiough notes that it is no coincidence

> ... that the main political celebration within the gay community each year, Gay/Lesbian Pride Week, commemorates a fight between gay people and police over a bar. ... that the gay liberation movement dates its beginning from that raid on the Stonewall bar. It is precisely because the bars have historically provided the bedrock on which gay culture is built that that raid takes on significance. (1980, p. 30)

A history of innovative music, dance drugs, and style amongst gay clubbers can be traced back to the 1970s and the 'golden days' of disco. The New York underground disco scene of the early 1970s was considered to have been predominantly gay, black and Hispanic and was fuelled by illicit consumption of drugs such as amphetamines, LSD and sedatives:

> ... gay culture helped shape disco – gave it much of its emotion and energy and sensuality; and those characteristics are more apparent now in a gay disco than in a straight one. (Riddiough, 1980, p. 18)

Reynolds echoes this view in his acknowledgement of the lineage from these gay disco roots to the British rave scene when he notes that 'rave's abandonment and demonstrativeness [was] ultimately derived from gay disco ...' (1997, p. 103).

Leading on from disco, the 1980s American house/garage scene was developed further by the black and gay communities, who as sexual and racial minorities were doubly excluded from white, heterosexist rock and pop. For example, in the 1980s Saturday nights at both the eponymous Chicago house club, the Warehouse, and the eponymous New York garage club, the Paradise Garage, were gay nights. Gay clubbers were also at the forefront of experimentation with illicit drugs in cities across the world from New York and San Francisco to Sydney, Ibiza, London and Amsterdam. Cocaine, amphetamines, LSD, PCP, methamphetamine (ice), poppers, cannabis and later ecstasy were all linked with gay dance scenes around the world. However, it was not simply the music and the recreational dance drug use which were seen to derive from the gay club scene. The whole bacchanalian revelry of the rave/dance party ethos, the hedonism in hard times and the open affection of 'luv'd up' clubbers were all in evidence in the gay club scene long before the 'decade of dance'. (Bacchus, or Dionysus, was known as the Lord of Dance, the God of Ecstasy, the ancient Greek god of ecstatic liberation, sensuality, wine and intoxication. His followers participated in ritualised activities involving music, dance, orgiastic sex and intoxicants to achieve altered states of consciousness.) Reynolds goes further in his analogies between the essence of dance culture and essence of gay culture. He suggests that the split in dance culture between finding/expressing oneself and losing control/losing oneself

> could be mapped on to the tension in gay culture between the politics of pride, unity and collective resilience, and the more hardcore 'erotic politics' of impersonal sexual encounters, 'deviant' practices and drugs. (1998, p. 22)

Furthermore, the very timing of the late 1980s rave/dance scene has been linked to a defining period in gay communities: the HIV/AIDS pandemic in Europe, North America and Australia (Lewis, 1994; Lewis and Ross, 1995; Saunders, 1995). The passionate pleasure seeking at dance parties is counterbalanced by the painful implications of the HIV/AIDS pandemic for individuals, gay communities and wider society. Many HIV-positive gay men became part of a stigmatised subculture within a stigmatised subculture, resulting in HIV-related stress, depression, and isolation alongside fears of invalidity and death. Historically and cross-culturally, ritualised behaviour such as dancing and the use of psycho-active substances have been linked to such periods of individual and community crisis. The intensity, hedonism and combination of spirituality and escapism in dance rituals has resulted in 'dances of death' across the centuries. (Echoed in the title of John Henry's (1992) article on medical complications of ecstasy use at British raves.) Group dancing has dual functions: as both a reaffirmation of individual identity and a reaffirmation of collective belonging, as a way of coping with pain and as a way of forgetting pain. Helman has noted that:

> Rituals are a feature of all human societies, large and small. They are an important part of the way that any social group celebrates, maintains and renews the world in which they live and the way they deal with dangers that threaten that world. (1990, p. 192, quoted in Lewis and Ross, 1995, p. 128)

Lewis and Ross draw parallels with historical 'dances of death' such as during Black Plague epidemics in twelfth- to eighteenth-century Europe which destroyed up to 25 per cent of the European population, and cross-cultural comparisons with dance rituals of urban Native American Indians who resumed tribal rituals in the twentieth century to help cope with alienating urban lifestyles (Lewis, 1994; Lewis and Ross, 1995). Lewis and Ross suggest that 'the dance party institution has provided many gay men with an adaptive social and psychological coping mechanism' (1995, p. 131).

Within the north-west of England, the history of dance club culture is also interwoven with the history of the gay club scene and in particular the development of Manchester's gay Village. The Village in Manchester, the largest outside London, flourished after the 1967 Sexual Offences Act decriminalised homosexuality for men aged 21 and over. Hindle (1994) estimates that on average a population of about 50,000 men aged 21 and over are needed to sustain each male or mixed gay venue in England or Wales. Whilst there are few gay venues in total in England and Wales, there are clusters in those cities which have large enough populations to sustain them at about 50,000:1, and also in smaller seaside resorts such as Blackpool, Brighton and Bournemouth which gays and lesbians travel to, rather than having substantial resident gay and lesbian communities. Hindle identified 23 gay venues in Manchester in mid-1993, divided into about half pubs/bars and about half dance clubs/discos, with their custom drawn from both Manchester residents and gay tourists from further afield. At the turn of the century this figure has probably doubled again.

Where gay venues develop they may become a physical, social and symbolic space for some gay men and lesbians:

> Gay bars ... provide the simplest safe social meeting place. ... They are probably the most important single feature of a gay community. (Hindle, 1994, p. 11)

Those gay men and lesbians who are 'out' at work and/or leisure may be amongst those who are physically out and about in pubs and clubs. There are issues of access, affordability and inclusion or exclusion to these city centre gay leisure spaces, however, with some lesbians and gays carving out lesbian and gay space elsewhere (Truman, forthcoming). This suggests that gay men and lesbians in the central leisure zones are likely to be a specific and unrepresentative minority within the gay minority. Jackson (1989) suggests that they are likely to be more vocal and politicised. It has been suggested that gay spaces, often in city centres, therefore have a dual purpose both for gays to 'come out' and as an economic, social and political focus for the gay and lesbian communities. They may also have negative implications as segregated gay 'ghettoes' with the 'push' factors of prejudice, discrimination, aggression and violence in the straight communities, not just the 'pull' factors of the gay space outlined above. Issues of safety, space and sexuality will be returned to in Chapter 6.

CONCLUSION

This chapter has provided an analysis of the writings of music journalists and popular commentators, academic researchers and first-hand observations by clubbers themselves of 1990s dance clubs and the ways in which they have been intersected by gender, race, socio-economic class and sexual orientation. We can see that claims have been made about the 1990s dance club as a 'new' social space in terms of social structure and inclusion of participants, both in contrast to earlier twentieth century dance halls and night clubs, and alternative contemporary licensed leisure locations such as pubs, bars and traditional night clubs. The relationship between social space – the dance club – social divisions and substance use is shown to have been a complex and dynamic process throughout the last decade.

Whilst there was evidence of new forms of social interaction and inclusion in the dance club regarding gender, socio-economic class and sexual orientation, this could not be considered the case with race, with the possible exception of jungle and the Asian underground. And the changes underway by the late 1990s eroded these embryonic features.

At the end of the 'decade of dance', acid house, rave and dance club culture has influenced both the post-rave dance music scene, with the plethora of sub-genres outlined in any current popular dance magazine, and the post-rave leisure scene, with more people from their early teens to their thirties involved in the clubbing/weekender lifestyle than ever. With the growing commercialisation and involvement of the licensed leisure trade, however, dance clubs in the late 1990s inevitably became more conservative, mainstream and conventional. Many of the utopian, spiritual and communal ideals of early dance club culture are now no more than an early 1990s memory reproduced at some 'old skool' and happy hardcore dance events.

So does the end of the 'decade of dance' mean the end of dance? British youth culture, with all the vibrancy and complexity of its sub-genres of music, fashion and style, is continually evolving and revolving, dividing and reforming. This has occurred throughout the second half of the last century and will continue into this new century. Whatever the form of entertainment, whatever the style of venue, there will continue to be demand for large public leisure spaces for people to take time out from 'work' – to relax, socialise, meet and make friends, listen to music, dance and consume a variety of food, drinks and psycho-active drugs. And with the extension of post-adolescence and young adulthood there is evidence of a broadening appeal of clubs. The licensed leisure industry has realised this appeal amongst the thirtysomethings, the so-called 'Peter Pan generation', who reach their mid-thirties but still want to go pubbing and clubbing, drink alcohol, possibly take drugs, meet sexual partners and have adventures. Perhaps the new millennium will see new challenges to the most embedded discrimination in clubland and one not discussed in this chapter, on the grounds of age.

This chapter has considered contemporary debate on British dance club culture, the socio-demographic profile of clubbers in clubland, and the ways in which gender, race, socio-economic class and sexual orientation shape club culture. In the next chapter we consider the composition of the sample of clubbers used in this study and the research methods used to acquire this sample from three north-west dance clubs.

3   Challenging Methods: Researching Clubs and Drugs from the Inside

Introduction

In this chapter we provide an overview of how we went about preparing for and setting up such a large-scale and innovative study. We purposefully adopt an informal style in this chapter both to help other researchers tune into how fieldwork inside busy, noisy night clubs can be undertaken but also so we can capture something of the every-night realities of club life.

We discuss how the three dance clubs were chosen and explore the characteristics of the clubs and their customer base as examples of dance music clubs. We then summarise how we trained our large fieldwork team and ensured their health and safety at work and maintained their night-time enthusiasm and productiveness in such demanding settings. We describe how the fieldwork, sampling, surveying and interviewing were undertaken and how through experience we learnt to adapt our strategies and practices to maximise effectiveness in encouraging clubbers to be monitored and even give urine samples.

We largely reached our targets, undertaking over 2,000 brief interviews with clubbers across 21 long fieldwork nights in three different dance clubs. We undertook in-depth interviews with 362 clubbers, collected over 200 voluntary urine samples from dance drug users, completed in-club intoxication and monitoring tests and ensured 54 dance drug users had detailed voluntary medical assessments at a later date. All this was completed without major incident, mishap or trouble of any sort thanks mainly to the reasonableness and co-operation of thousands of clubbers – a salutary point in itself given the negative media and public constructions of clubland.

Setting up the project

Developing protocols

After some fruitless discussion with the Department of Health and the Medical Research Council for whom assessing 'health' in clubland seemed a research and political step too far, this project was funded by the Economic and Social Research Council. The sponsor's expert referees, whilst genuinely encouraging, warned however that we were on an over-ambitious, high-risk (ad)venture and should not be expected to meet all our goals and objectives. We were equally apprehensive given the paucity of other studies and the tendency for what investigations had been undertaken to rely on interviewing clubbers outside clubland. Seasoned club goers and watchers smiled knowingly at our 'unrealistic' plans to collect urine samples from 'pissed up–drugged up' customers.

From such apprehension came a commitment to prepare for, plan and pilot our fieldwork with great care, paying much attention to the fine detail and hopefully having a strategy for every worst contingency – from being caught in a police raid to having an interviewer assaulted.

Our proposals were assessed by local Medical Ethics Committees and accepted as appropriate. We adopted the 'informed consent' procedures they recommended, especially for obtaining the volunteers for the medical assessments of 54 dance drug users at a University medical facility. We liaised extensively with the police, meeting with licensing officers, plain-clothes and serious crime–drug squad managers. Our interview team, at their request, all had criminal record searches to check they didn't have drugs convictions. The clean bill of health ensured the police felt able to support our work, thus avoiding any problems as and when they inspected or raided clubs which we were working in. We also liaised with local authority officials (licensing, community safety) and a local drugs agency with a strong commitment to providing information and advice to clubbers.

During these negotiations we also obtained opinions and views from all these key players about their perspectives on the dance club–night club scene in Greater Manchester. The politics of drugs and clubs were very potent and often quite tense between these different professional groups. Disagreements revolving around the operation of inter-agency partnerships and the conflicting priorities between law enforcement and creating a lively 24-hour leisure scene were central to this debate. Once all the negotiations were complete we set about negotiating with club owners/managers to choose our three fieldwork clubs.

The three clubs

We have already discussed how the diversification and commercialisation of 'dance' and associated musical genres during the 1990s make the classification of different types of dance clubs and night clubs very difficult. The diversity found amongst several thousand clubs around the country makes the chances of us ever having wholly representative research data practically zero. Our focus on dance clubs – clubs which played variations of late 1990s dance music – whilst reducing the universe from which to sample, still meant that whatever the merits of our choices, we would not be able to demonstrate broader representiveness.

To illustrate this we looked at one large city in north-west England and its complete list of venues with full, provisional and pending public entertainment licenses at the end of 1997. The total was 262. However the majority of these venues were not night clubs or dance clubs, but hotels, pubs, café bars and social clubs that, whilst they may hold discos and dance nights, had other multiple entertainment functions even though licensed in a way consistent with being a night club. In fact only 43 were identifiable as 'night clubs' which held regular youth-oriented music and dance events as a primary function. And of these only 11 were, in our professional opinion, specifically recognisable as dance clubs, the remainder playing mainly pop, rock and 'indie' music.

It is patently clear therefore that once we move beyond common-sense definitions of 'night clubs' and attempt a more scientific classification we find a very slippery concept. Our concentration on dance clubs is because they are the target of public and political concern about young people and ecstasy use. We could attempt to make the case for our three venues being representative of the region's dance club venues but it would be contentious and once we move to 'night club' representativeness any claims would be ill-conceived. In short, the only goal of representativeness we could realistically strive for was that our research respondents were representative of clubbers at each venue. We will describe whether this was achieved at the end of the chapter.

Several other considerations affected club choice. We selected sizeable venues to ensure we could achieve the large sample sizes we wished to generate within the resource limits set. This ruled out small clubs with only a few hundred capacity. We also wanted to have three rather different clubs illustrating the diversity found in the dance club sector, as discussed in the previous chapter. After the extensive liaisons with the key players discussed earlier and attending prospective clubs as customers, three clubs were chosen to be approached. All were within tolerable travelling distance of our domestic and professional bases.

Each of the three clubs we approached agreed to co-operate with the research. We cannot be sure of why they immediately did so given that whilst we emphasised the 'health' agenda we made no secret of the drugs agenda. It may well be that seeing the status of our research, endorsed by key players (e.g. the police, local authority) they had no wish to cross, they felt that this would be to their advantage as 'responsible' club owners/managers. Our overall impression however was that our research was seen as worthwhile, well organised and non-threatening given that we guaranteed to disguise the clubs' identities.

The Warehouse club was set in a former factory/warehouse complex in the city centre. It was a multi-level venue with a large outdoor cobbled courtyard which was an integral feature of the club. Customers entered the club at one end of the courtyard. Doors to reception, cloakroom, bars and dance floors were located at the other end.

The City Centre club was also a multi-level venue renowned for its design features. The entrance to this club was at ground level straight off a main street. On the ground floor was a main dance floor and bar but the club had two more levels with a second dance floor, bar, food hatch and toilets on the middle level and a further bar and dance floor on the top level.

The Leisure Centre was a very large single-level leisure centre which was trans-formed into a dance venue at weekends thanks to impressive feats of interior construction, scaffolding and electrical engineering. A complex in its own grounds with extensive car parking, the Leisure Centre had a canopied entrance into a reception area which led off to a very large arena and thoroughfare to toilets, food counter, large bar with lounge and, for popular dance events, two more large arenas. This venue had wheelchair access and thus wheelchair-using dancers.

Each club represented a different dance music genre. The Leisure Centre played hardcore, old skool and happy hardcore music, developing out of 1990s 'rave' music. The Warehouse club hosted a variety of different dance, jungle and techno nights with nationally renowned DJs and the City Centre club played mainly house music. These musical distinctions were related to the customer base. The Warehouse club had the highest percentage of students in higher education and Black and Asian customers, the Leisure Centre had a younger 'working class', employed clientele and the City Centre club had a slightly older customer base with substantial higher education representation and a strong gay/lesbian and bisexual clientele particularly at weekends. The two city centre clubs would routinely have several hundred customers on Thursday/Friday/Saturday nights and the Leisure Centre would entertain up to two thousand clubbers at Saturday night dance events.

The key to successfully completing the fieldwork in each of these clubs was adaptability. The specific architecture and layout of these venues, the 'flow' of clubbers, the siting of toilets, chill out areas, bars, food sales and sound sources were set and we thus had to adapt our approach, the siting of our work station and so on to these realities. We will illustrate all this as we discuss typical fieldwork nights. The key methodological or technical point is that one must assess the club both empty and full and plan where different research tasks are best, or often least worst, carried out bearing in mind supervisory and health and safety responsibilities and the need to be able to hear respondents' replies whilst also affording them some privacy.

The fieldwork foundations

The grand plan

Figure 3.1 is an overview of the types of samples we created with the numbers achieved. The idea was to conduct sweep surveys representative of the clubbers at the venue over seven nights at each club. From the *club sample* we isolated two other samples for detailed interviews: the *comparison* sample who were not taking dance drugs on the night in question and had not done so for two years and the *dance drugs* sample who had and were. Finally from the dance drug interviewees we selected volunteers for a medical assessment at a university facility at a later date.

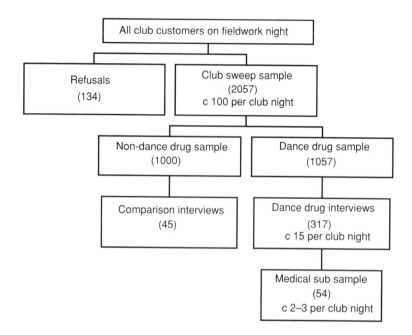

Figure 3.1   The samples and their size

We had three key schedules for administering inside the clubs: the brief sweep survey, the dance drug users' interview and monitoring schedule and the non-dance drug using comparisons' interview schedule. The sweep survey was on two sides of A4 paper containing 14 questions. It was administered by the fieldwork team. It was intended to collect a maximum of information in a minimum period of time; typically, between one and two minutes, and as a result of extensive piloting, it was carefully phrased for comprehension and conversational flow. Demographic questions included gender, race and sexual orientation. Gender was visually assessed and recorded by the interviewer. Both race and sexual orientation were assessed through self-definition by respondents during the interview. The questions were phrased: 'Would you describe yourself as black, white, Asian, or other?' and 'Would you describe yourself as straight, gay/lesbian or bisexual?' We were and remain aware of the limitations of asking these questions in the way that we did, particularly in public leisure settings. These issues, however, were balanced by the centrality of race, gender, and sexual orientation to our theoretical concerns as social researchers, by their relationship with the specific subject of dance club culture as we have seen in the last chapter, and by the need to obtain this information in the quickest and most accurate way possible, causing the least confusion or offence to respondents. In fact, missing data on these questions was very low: only two respondents on the race question (0.1 per cent) and four on the sexual orientation question (0.2 per cent). We suspected, however, in the City Centre club that a proportion of customers who were actually 'straight' or heterosexual had claimed to be bisexual at this club because they were concerned about admission to the club with its door policy on Friday and Saturday nights specifying gay men and lesbians and their straight friends. Co-ordinator fieldwork notes illustrate:

> Three young men arrived together, and Craig took one, me another, and Fiona the third (very drunk) one. Craig and I were standing fairly near to one another when doing the sweep, so I could hear some of their sweep interview. When we got to the sexual orientation question, both my sweepee and Craig's said they were 'bisexual'. Later, Craig told me he doubted they were bisexual and thought they had assumed we were affiliated with the club in some way and that they would be denied access if they said they were straight. He was right about this – both later admitted when interviewed that this was why they answered the way they did. (Co-ordinator fieldwork notes)

Although we expended considerable effort to make clear to potential interviewees that we were not working as part of the club management, it is inevitable that some customers will nevertheless have suspected that admitting to being straight may have resulted in expulsion from the club. Over the course of the seven nights' fieldwork in the City Centre club, we found that occasionally sweep interviewees later admitted to having stated they were bisexual though they considered themselves to be straight. Thus, we should expect that a considerable proportion that we did not 'find out' about will have done the same. Bearing this in mind, the proportion of bisexual respondents in the club sample was higher at the City Centre club (13.0 per cent) than in the other two clubs (2.8 per cent and 1.1 per cent).

We are disappointed with the lack of valid data on the category 'bisexual', but our approach in analysing results by sexual orientation nevertheless has been to present data for respondents who indicated their sexual orientation to be bisexual, but to concentrate discussion on comparisons between respondents describing themselves as 'gay/lesbian' and straight.

The interview schedules were longer and more complex than the sweep surveys, with typical administration times of over 30 minutes. The comparison schedule for non-current/recent dance drug users had the same structure and content as the dance drug schedule but with some additional questions about triggers/temptations to use dance drugs, reasons for not taking them and perceptions of clubbers who did.

The dance drug schedule began with a section on 'clubbing': regularity of attendance, likes and dislikes, types of music, importance as a leisure activity and money spent.

The next section aimed to build up a comprehensive drugs history including tobacco and alcohol. From here the schedule focussed on current drug use and 'tonight's' drug use and the reasons for taking drugs. The next theme was about 'risk', negative effects of drugs, the scale and nature of any recovery period and previous drug-related cautions/convictions. The interviewees were then asked about their health and any possibly drug-related health problems and subsequent help seeking. The final sections focussed on safety and security and how clubbers obtained, exchanged and took their drugs and how they planned to get home.

Creating the interview sample

Of the listed drugs in the brief sweep interview five were used as part of the criteria for developing the comparison and dance drug samples. These five drugs were *amphetamines, ecstasy, LSD, cocaine powder* and *crack cocaine*. All have been variously associated with the term 'dance drug' by other researchers. Crack cocaine may appear an unlikely dance floor drug but it was associated with some mid-1990s jungle clubs (Saunders, 1997; Headon, 1994) and was thus included for reasons of comprehensiveness. In fact, although 142 respondents in the club sweep sample had ever tried crack (7 per cent), only three respondents (0.1 per cent) either planned to or had taken it on the fieldwork night.

We are also aware that other drugs, such as cannabis, poppers or GHB, are used in the context of the dance club. We did not include use of these other drugs as criteria for eligibility in the dance drug sample for a number of reasons, and we now discuss some of these. In relation to cannabis, as an example, research suggests that the prevalence of cannabis use is widespread and in fact it is the most commonly used illegal drug in Britain. To include such an extensively used drug would cast our net widely and perhaps indiscriminately. If it had been included as a criterion dance drug, cannabis users would have dominated the sample to the exclusion of users of other dance drugs. Secondly, the use of cannabis is not specific to the context of the dance club, although it is used there. For example, respondents in Release's survey (1997) reported that the most popular drug taken in clubs was ecstasy, but that the most popular drug to take generally was cannabis. Cannabis is widely consumed by young people at home, at parties, in public spaces, parks and the streets, as well as pubs and clubs (Measham et al., 1998a). Therefore, although cannabis might be used in clubs, or indeed after attendance at clubs as a key 'chill out' drug, it is rarely considered to be a dance drug as such. Our reasoning also relates, thirdly, to its psycho-active effects. Cannabis is often classed as a depressant whereas dance drugs can be categorised as either stimulants in the case of amphetamines, ecstasy, crack and cocaine or hallucinogenic in the case of LSD. We also excluded the occasionally used 'deliriants' such as ketamine and GHB (gamma-hydroxy-butyrate) as key dance drugs although as we shall see they were used by some of our respondents.

The *dance drug* sample was constructed from all those sweep respondents or 'sweepees' who:

- had taken at least one of the five key dance drugs in the past three months
- and also reported having already imbibed or planned to take a dance drug when briefly interviewed on the night in question.

We can, in retrospect, review our dance drug inclusion–exclusion criteria by looking at their sample's recent drugs histories. Table 3.1 shows how many more of the sweepees would have been included as dance drug users if we had not set a three-month recency threshold but merely required a previous (to the fieldwork night) lifetime experience of one of the five dance drugs.

Table 3.1   Effects of three-month criterion on dance drug sample: past three months and less frequent

	Dance Drug Sample (Tonight & past 3 months)	Irregular Users (Tonight & prior to past 3 months)
Amphetamines	636 (97.4)	17 (2.6)
Ecstasy	718 (96.8)	24 (1.1)
LSD	41 (89.1)	5 (10.9)
Cocaine	134 (95.7)	6 (4.3)
Crack	3 (100.0)	

As we can see opening this gate would in fact only bring in small numbers. The vast majority of sweep interviewees dancing on drugs (n = 1,057) on any fieldwork night had also consumed a dance drug at least once in the past three months. Moreover, based on the interview samples only (n = 362), we found nearly nine out of ten had used ecstasy and amphetamines (less so LSD) in the past month as well. This suggests our criteria were reasonable and that the results would not have altered greatly had we modified the drugs history inclusion–exclusion criteria. Clubbers who are dance drug users are, in the main, regular users.

The *comparison sample* was selected from all those sweep interviewees who had not taken a dance drug in the past two years and who had not and did not intend to do so on the fieldwork night. These interviews were conducted by one of the co-ordinators using the relevant schedule. As we shall see in due course, although dance drug free on the night and for the past two years, the comparison sample was in fact also very drug experienced and a long way away from the traditional notions of an abstentious control group.

Creating the medical assessment sub sample

We attempted to recruit two or three volunteers from the dance drug interview sample created on each fieldwork night to attend a full medical assessment at a commercial facility at Manchester University geared to undertake physical and medical assessments (the results of which are discussed in Chapter 5). We had fairly detailed 'packs' for these volunteers including standardised informed consent pro formas. We almost certainly 'excluded' dance drug interviewees who were very intoxicated from this exercise, ducking the dilemmas of whether a seriously E'd up clubber is often too compliant, once a rapport has developed, to give sober informed consent. Each volunteer received travel costs and a £30 music voucher.

Quota sampling and sub sampling

Perhaps in retrospect our attempts to systematically sample venue entrants to produce representativeness of the customer base and to quota sample 1:1 by gender and 1:9 black/Asian to white customers to ensure these key variables could be effectively analysed, was over-ambitious. We will refer to the strengths and weaknesses of this in due course. In terms of describing how the sub samples were created – this was done by each fieldworker. From their sweep interviewees, perhaps 10–15 per night, they would select two or three who fitted the dance drug sample criteria and if these respondents agreed to participate then these clubbers became their responsibility both to interview but also to track and encourage to see the nurse for monitoring and give a urine sample.

This process was repeated to create the medical sub sample in that when the fieldworkers interviewed a dance drug user who fitted the criteria and was also willing to give informed consent (and thus their name and address unlike other respondents), they would ask the respondent to attend a medical.

The fieldwork team

We recruited nine temporary interviewers and a nurse to work alongside the three lead researchers. This 'pool' gave us some flexibility over the size of the fieldwork team on any one night so we could adapt to venue and event size and give people the odd weekend 'off' given we worked over 21 fieldwork nights. Our ideal interviewer would be experienced in social research, comfortable in a dark and noisy dance club, capable of obtaining highly sensitive information from strangers, be able to encourage clubbers to take time out for a detailed interview, and submit to pulse, temperature and intoxication tests and give a urine sample. In the absence of comprehensive previous experience (which few of us had!) we selected those with interview experience with young people and familiarity and empathy with the club scene. They were extensively trained and also learnt 'on the job' during the piloting and initial nights of fieldwork. Of the team three were gay/lesbian, one was British-born black and one disabled; six were men and six were women and all but one were in their twenties and thirties.

All the interviewers passed police vetting procedures. They were familiarised with the Misuse of Drugs Act. They were expected to remain sober and not to be under the influence of illicit drugs during working hours. They were permitted to consume up to four units of alcohol over the four to eight hours of a fieldwork night. Interviewers were asked to dress in clean, presentable and modest clothes and encouraged to fit in as far as possible with the appearance of customers in each of the three clubs. Each wore a University of Manchester photo identification card and carried a clipboard. Each was issued with a personal alarm but in practice the fieldworkers chose to discard these as they quickly felt safe and secure. Finally, once fieldwork began elaborate procedures were set in place such as a contract with a private hire minibus/taxi firm to ensure safe travel arrangements.

Working in clubs

Piloting

Although we had a formal piloting period this was, in retrospect, part of an on-going process of adaptation. Given the differences between the clubs in terms of size, layout, customer base and so on, there was always a sense of reflection and reflexivity, particularly in respect of organisational and administrative arrangements.

After several initial drafts of the three schedules to be used in the clubs, they were piloted in the City Centre club (to which we returned several months later as our third fieldwork club). Piloting of these instruments occurred over the course of four fieldwork nights. The schedules were redrafted after the first two fieldwork nights, and again after piloting was complete. The sweep interview schedule was also revised after piloting, changing, for example, the order of questions to improve the flow of the interview. We also decided to record an interviewer assessment of gender and race of all those who refused to do a sweep, to obtain some data on refusals in order to assess how representative the eventual club sample would be.

Prior to piloting, we had anticipated that it would be possible to approach every 'n'th customer entering the club ('n' varying each night depending upon expected numbers), in order to obtain a representative sample of customers entering the club. However, during the piloting we realised that this procedure would be impractical for a number of reasons. Firstly, customers tended to enter the club in large, social groupings and quickly disperse to other areas. Singling out one potential sweepee from a group of friends was problematic. Either friends would hang around unoccupied or gather round the sweep interview. Sometimes we were mistaken for club staff and approached by clubbers with club-related queries. We also found our initial 'singling out' approach as customers entered clubs encouraged refusals. We thus adapted both our timing and strategy so that we approached clubbers as they were 'settling in', waiting for friends to reappear from cloakrooms and toilets, or first walking around the venue. We also used two or three sweepers simultaneously to overcome the problem of 'singling out' by allowing a cluster of sweep interviews to be undertaken simultaneously. We stuck to this approach throughout the fieldwork and continued to adhere to our gender and race quotas.

Updating the fieldworkers

Originally it was planned to send updates to the fieldworkers by post during the first week or two between work nights to respond to teething troubles in the fieldwork. In fact this became a continuous weekly feature, written by the co-ordinators and posted to team members. A short team meeting prior to starting fieldwork was built around these memos. The agenda focussed on the quality of each fieldworker's weekly returns, discussion of the previous session's work, fieldwork observations and thoughts on how well the interviews (which had to be completed appropriately and returned within a few days) had gone. There were also items about research procedures, quota sampling, exact transport arrangements and so on. This updating also helped fieldworkers who had been rested or missed a weekend to refocus. The latent function of all this was to provide encouragement and engender a sense of professionalism and team work whereby team members took responsibility for one another and the success of the overall process.

Developing effective relationships with clubbers

We discussed the importance of being flexible and adaptive earlier. Rather than describe all this for each club we illustrate the kinds of processes we adopted, the point being that any other researchers will have different problems and contingencies to face but will be well served by making careful on-going assessments and adapting and thus improving performance within the constraints imposed by clubland. We illustrate this in respect of how we came to utilise a *work station* in each club and how we 'negotiated' difficult or sensitive moments when interacting with clubbers.

We had originally anticipated that each interviewer having undertaken their sweep interviews would then, having identified three or four in-depth interview subjects, be responsible for relocating them and negotiating an interview time and visit to our nurse for monitoring and to get their urine bottle to take to the toilets. We learnt quite quickly that a work station could become the hub of the whole fieldwork night and that a good proportion of dance drug sample interviewees would come/return to us if we were effectively sited (e.g. near chill out areas, toilets, visible from main thoroughfares). This realisation arose from work in the Warehouse, our first club, as these fieldwork notes illustrate.

The geography of the club worked better than I'd thought for both the sweep and the interviews. The sweeps can be conducted when people are queuing by the metal crowd-control barricades to get in, and there's enough room to take them to one side, or else after they've paid and they've come back out to put their coats in the cloakroom. Then the courtyard is also the best and most obvious place to conduct the interviews. Later on in the warm summer evening it becomes a natural 'chill out' area and some people even continue to dance on the two little podiums outside. Others sit on the sides of the podiums and up the first two or three steps of the fire escape. It's cool and quiet enough for people to take a bit of a break and be interviewed. Some people want to come outside anyway so don't see it as a hardship being dragged away from the club, especially if all their mates have come outside as well. (Co-ordinator fieldwork notes)

And again:

Courtyard got packed with 70 to 90 people later on, lots being swept and interviewed. Others sitting down and chilling out. Our cool box/bags/sweets/cigs/chewing gum 'work station' has become a bit of a hub. This lets people come out and find us if they've agreed to be interviewed and are keen enough. I've found that the drinkers are less willing to come out and find me to be interviewed for the comparison. It also lets people come and ask us further questions about the research – to clarify exactly who we are and what we're doing. (Co-ordinator fieldwork notes)

The key point is that paying attention to the fine detail and continuously responding to it in shaping the fieldwork approach in each club, sometimes even in respect of different crowds on different nights, is vital. Free chewing gum and sweets in plastic tubs on the front of our work station for instance, an apparently tiny detail, made an enormous difference to our image, to clubbers talking informally with us, indeed to trusting us. Clubbers on stimulant dance drugs often find they need to chew: thus any researchers tuned into this insider knowledge, and concerned with clubbers' health and welfare might be considered OK by them. We also pinned posters around the club and in the toilets explaining who we were, our independence from both the police and the club and our 'health of clubbers' agenda, which appeared effective. This 'relationship' can be built on: the research team are in the club each week, they're friendly, hard working, even get on the dance floor for the last half an hour of the event, my mate's been interviewed, the paramedics talk with them, the bouncers and bar staff 'accept' them.

This move from scepticism (are they anything to do with the police?) to tolerance to co-operation is important. It helped keep the sample representative in that 'refusers' in week one can become participants by week five for instance. On the other hand, it leads to difficulties for the research process with people 'volunteering' to be interviewed or have physical assessments by the nurse, and groups of mates gathering around an interviewee and listening to and 'contributing' to answers. We had completely 'out of it' clubbers coming to the work station and sitting down in the hopes of a philosophical debate or if they were drunk, a verbal scrap about the merits of different research techniques by which our accumulated research experience is dismissed with one misquote of Durkheim!

Many of our on-the-spot encounters with clubbers were humorous but nevertheless had the potential to go wrong and cause embarrassment or disagreement. Again our point is that the fieldwork team had to be continuously tuned in to the venue, event and the social interactions involved. For example at the sweep whilst each interviewer utilised the self-definition question to record race (would you describe yourself as Black, white, Asian or other?) and sexual orientation (would you describe yourself as straight, gay/lesbian or bisexual?), gender was visually assessed by the interviewer. This normally straightforward process is occasionally challenged in clubland as this fieldwork co-ordinator's note illustrates:

> Interesting/embarrassing gender dilemmas for researchers. The very first sweep question is male/female boxes, which we tick but it hasn't been obvious a couple of times tonight. So what do you do? Just close your eyes and tick a box? You CAN'T ask them! Tony put someone down on the sweep as a man and she saw this and said no she was a woman. I swept a very very pretty 17-year-old with a girly made-up face and shaved head with leopard spots, but utterly flat-chested in a skin-tight tee-shirt, so on balance probably a boy. Also s/he had a very high-pitched, natural effeminate voice. I left the gender question and moved swiftly onto the others hoping for clues. But in the sexual orientation question, s/he said s/he was bisexual and has a boyfriend, so no clues there. Debbie also had experiences of the 'third way', the new categories invented by respondents at the City Centre club, e.g. a man said he wasn't homosexual, heterosexual or bisexual, he was just 'sexual'. And a Black man refused to define his race, saying he was of the 'human race'. My initial impression is the City Centre club crowd is largely older, more wised-up and has more critical awareness of language than at the other two clubs. (Co-ordinator fieldwork notes)

Dealing with the decibels

A serious concern, even objection, to researching inside dance clubs and night clubs is that the music is too loud to allow meaningful social interaction. Friends and partners can put their mouths in each other's ears to make themselves heard but this intimacy is not the norm when interviewing strangers. In choosing large venues we incidentally gave ourselves much greater chance of finding quieter areas to set up our work station and find similar space for the detailed interviews. In selecting the clubs and first visiting them on busy nights we had to be convinced that the decibels would not drown out the interview conversation. Undoubtedly there will be clubs, particularly smaller venues, where fieldwork is impractical. This is yet another reason why full representativeness in clubland will never be achieved.

This said, there are few genuinely quiet areas in functioning clubs and hearing every word the interviewee utters is not always possible. We dealt with this by ensuring our interviewers wrote up their interviews within a couple of days of each fieldwork night and distinguished between exact 'quotes' and the thrust of an answer or detailed response. For this reason we, unusually, often include fieldworkers' interpretations of an exchange or response in place of direct quotes. For example:

> When you are so intoxicated by ecstasy you see people wearing glasses everywhere, not normal glasses, sparkly ones. It makes him really giggle to himself and feel excited. One guy told him he sees people going round with cups of tea. That seemed even weirder. (Based on interview 210501)

> She doesn't go clubbing much now she's stopped taking drugs. She doesn't see the point, though she misses the dancing. She does think though that 'drug' clubs are nicer places to be than 'alcohol' clubs because of the good atmosphere and lack of aggression. (Based on interview 010105)

Interviewing the intoxicated and vulnerable

As we shall see in the next chapter, the majority of clubbers will, certainly by one or two o'clock in the morning, be varyingly intoxicated either by alcohol, drugs or most often a mixture of both. They may also be very tired and thus less thoughtful or accurate in conversation. There were some respondents who we regarded as potentially unsuitable for recruitment to the interview samples by the time we'd finished the sweep with them. We also had interviewees who 'lost it' over the course of the fieldwork night in terms of being alert or focussed enough to be regarded as reliable informants. Clearly there are some subjective judgements to be made here although the dance drug sample undertook intoxication tests (see Chapter 5). We can only warn of this issue and note that our own remedy was to make shared, on the spot judgements:

> He was willing to be interviewed but we had to abandon the interview after 20 minutes as he was tripping and finding it impossible to think ... his vision was severely disrupted, everything splitting into eight and dancing round in circles. (171110)

She happily snogged my previous interviewee when he came over – they did some 'drug bonding' because he knew what the interview was about so they talked about how fabulous ecstasy was. I had to keep sending him off so I could finish the interview. (021114)

At this point in the interview she was feeling the effects of the speed and the ecstasy she had taken. She insisted on going to dance and said she would return to finish the interview in about an hour. Unfortunately she did not return. (010406)

This was not a very pleasant interview for me. The man was drunk and had earlier said was only here to get laid. He made suggestive and sexual comments a lot during the interview (e.g. what other drugs are you planning to take tonight 'pussy'?). He talked about his sex drive and his 'dick' (much of which I faithfully wrote into the schedule). He was swinging from interested to really quite annoyed at the fact he was being interviewed at all. (151111)

Whilst we felt that with experience we could tell whether respondents were mainly drinking, were on amphetamines or cocaine, or ecstasy by their demeanour and verbal style even before gathering the data, an important ethical issue needs discussing. Neither the medical ethics committees nor the researchers had fully addressed the issue of informed consent whilst under the influence of dance drugs and alcohol. Our impression by the end of the fieldwork was that the ecstasy users may have been disproportionately co-operative, even compliant, in respect of agreeing to be interviewed, monitored, and give a urine sample (although as we shall see later in this chapter, ecstasy users were no more likely than non-users to agree to be interviewed, and in fact, respondents who had consumed more alcohol were more amenable to being interviewed). During the fieldwork we took care not to abuse such compliance and those agreeing to a full medical assessment for instance were recontacted and asked to reaffirm consent over the following week. However there is a real issue here in respect of informed consent and intoxication when conducting in situ research which needs to form part of future ethical considerations in this type of research.

A further difficulty with interviewing alcohol-/drug-affected clubbers is that they sometimes become emotional or distressed as they find themselves talking of unresolved worries or issues. We will deal with the broader issue of their psychological states in Chapter 5. Here it is sufficient to mention that there were some painful and poignant interviews and several which troubled the interviewers. Occasionally we switched roles whereupon completing our research tasks we offered advice or referral, given that several of the team were professionally qualified so to do.

At several points in the interview she seemed to feel affected by the interview itself – it seemed to bring her down a bit when she realised the extent of her drug history or thought about the future. 'I've never sat down and thought about it like this.' (060302)

Although he was willing to talk he seemed withdrawn/low on occasions – looking back at his interview schedule he possibly felt the need to share some of his 'down' experiences of drugs and possibly the interview was an outlet. As we talked more it became apparent that although he was sociable there were underlying issues/feelings he wouldn't raise. In a rush of openness he admitted that speed had led him to contemplate suicide and the depression (which he appeared to have sought no help for) lasted for at least six months. This is obviously still a concern for him because in the future he suggests there may be psychological problems. I couldn't find him after the interview. He was certainly the most intense of the three interviews. He told me of his daily speed habit which he uses intravenously. Dave knew he needed help and had been to various doctors, drop-ins and drug teams ... it was at this point my social conscience wrestled with my purely research role. Fiona and I agreed that Tina in her capacity as a drugs worker should talk to him. Tonight I saw drug use from a different angle ... I really hope he gets some help. Soon. (180908)

Medical observations

Although in general our procedures for monitoring the pulse rate, temperature, pupil dilation and intoxication of our dance drug sample went fairly well, the realities of clubland did intrude. The procedures were undertaken by our nurse. Two infra-red ear thermometers were purchased for use by the fieldwork nurse to measure the body temperature of dance drug respondents and a comparison group of 45 interviewed clubbers who had not taken dance drugs on the fieldwork night. These thermometers measured the infra-red heat generated by the eardrum and surrounding tissue (the ear's temperature is very similar to the temperature control centre in the brain because its blood supply is very close to the brain). The fieldwork nurse performed these tasks with medical professionalism and this no doubt added to the fact that no respondents refused to have medical observations carried out. The authority and ease with which the nurse conducted these tests helped to override feelings of concern about invasion of personal space, in particular being touched by a stranger.

The use of the thermometer was not without difficulties, however. The accuracy of thermometer readings and the relevance of the results will be discussed further in Chapter 5. It is worth noting here, however, that the thermometers proved more erratic than at first anticipated, particularly in the Warehouse club in which observations were conducted outdoors in the courtyard:

The weather was much cooler last night with regular drizzles of rain and odd spitting. It was so cool outside in the courtyard that both thermometers wouldn't work. Apparently it has to be over 16 degrees Celsius for them to work properly. The nurse had to keep both thermometers down his trousers pockets between use and that seemed to work. But he felt like a cowboy with a big gun in each holster! (Co-ordinator fieldwork notes)

There was also the issue of timing of temperatures. We decided to conduct medical observations after the in-depth interview was completed, to allow the respondent 30 minutes or so to relax and get to know the interviewer and the purpose of the research. Leaving the observations until after the interview made sense from the perspective of developing rapport in the research process, but caused its own difficulties, again in the Warehouse club in which observations were conducted outdoors in the courtyard:

The nurse commented regarding people's temperatures that if they came straight out of the club it was higher than normal. But for most of our dance drug interviewees their temperature was taken at the end of the interview, after 20 to 30 minutes of sitting outside in the cool, quietly talking, and this gave them plenty of time to chill out and their temperature to return more or less to normal. (Co-ordinator fieldwork notes)

Other challenges orbited around taking the pulse of people who have taken dance drugs – the pulse is often weak, intermittent or irregular. There is quite an art to taking the pulse, particularly in loud dance clubs with music of 150 beats per minute or more, which distracts from accurate counting of a weak or irregular pulse. The fieldwork co-ordinators also on occasion had to take pulse and ear temperatures and therefore had to develop some competence. It was only then that we fully realised the special skills required for this task:

I felt fairly confident about the pulses: as before, most were fairly easy to do, and a minority quite difficult, and this night two were difficult. This happens particularly when someone has had a lot of speed or ecstasy, and they appear quite 'off it'. The pulse then can be faint and quite irregular. The other problem is that respondents also have difficulty staying still, and small 'tensing' in the wrist means that tendons pop up and down, interfering with feeling the pulse. (Co-ordinator fieldwork notes)

Interestingly, both club customers and club staff who were not involved in our research came up to the nurse and asked for their temperature or pulse to be taken for personal interest or reassurance.

Respondents' pupils were assessed as being either dilated or not dilated as a further indicator of stimulant drug use. There were also difficulties with this, however, as people who had not had stimulant drugs sometimes had dilated pupils because of being in a dark environment. Conversely, those who had had stimulant drugs, when standing in bright environments, sometimes experienced a loss of pupil dilation. In fact, most of the sample of dance drug interviewees (88.7 per cent) had dilated pupils, and the proportion was unrelated to which drugs interviewees had consumed.

Collecting urine samples from interviewees proved to be a challenge that we met with considerable success. As no other drugs researchers to our knowledge have ever attempted to collect urine samples within a club environment, we had no basis on which to estimate what level of compliance would be obtained. Indeed, colleagues, police officers and drugs agency staff all were adamant that this plan was too ambitious. There were several reasons for their pessimism. First, and perhaps most significant, was the legal issue: it is one thing for interview respondents to self-report and even have recorded their illicit drug use, but urine samples move one step further by providing objective verification of the ingestion of illegal substances, and potential material evidence for criminal conviction. The second problem was the practicality of requesting and obtaining urine. Our plan, to ask strangers in clubs to provide urine samples in small pots in the club toilets, was seen to be impractical, bizarre, perhaps even perverted. Colleagues warned that we might be endangering ourselves and our team by even making such a request. Thirdly, there were gender-related issues of how to collect the urine. Whilst there were some amused appraisals of men's aiming ability under the influence of alcohol or drugs, the practicalities of women's aiming ability was seriously discussed with medical advisors, along with the possibility of providing extra funnel equipment for them. After extensive inquiries into the range of specimen pot shapes and sizes on offer, we used a pot with a diameter of 50 millimetres which we felt most women would realistically be able to use. As we discuss below, however, inevitably there were spills by both respondents and researchers. Fourthly, it was anticipated that there would be a high refusal rate. Club goers may well agree to spend some of their night being interviewed, even about their drug use, but could balk at the suggestion that they provide us with a urine specimen – the collection of body fluids is not a typical part of anyone's leisure time activities. Club goers may further have wondered whether a request for a urine sample meant that interviewers disbelieved their self-report answers and were seeking some sort of verification.

However, in spite of these concerns and misgivings, we successfully obtained 222 of 317 potential urine samples, a success rate of over two-thirds. In fact all of the 317 respondents in the interview dance drug sample from whom we requested urine samples initially consented to providing urine. Of those who eventually did not provide samples, only a small number did not do so because they had changed their minds (24, 6.6 per cent). Of the remainder, 20 (5.5 per cent) 'couldn't go' (due to the production of urine being restricted by being dehydrated in the club and/or the influence of dance drugs); the rest (50, 15.8 per cent) had lost the motivation to return their specimen pot, having become further engrossed in their enjoyment of the night, or occasionally returned their sample after the fieldworkers had finished work.

One man did a (urine) sample and said it was knocked out of his hand by a bloke pushing open his cubicle door before he'd put the top on and he didn't feel able or willing to bother again. (Co-ordinator fieldwork notes)

However, on the other hand:

The level of co-operation and commitment to the research by some of the clubbers is heartwarming and quite incredible. Last week one young woman was dehydrated and couldn't provide a urine sample. She took away the pot and said she'd try later. One and a half hours elapsed and we were waiting outside for the taxi home, and we'd written her off. But at 2.30am. she came bounding up to us with her sample, past all the door staff and the whole research team, clutching her urine pot in her hand – making a total of 15 samples for the night. (Co-ordinator fieldwork notes)

Members of the research team reported increasing confidence in asking clubbers to provide urine samples after the first fieldwork night. There was an initial feeling amongst the fieldworkers that such a request was brazen, making them feel awkward and uncomfortable, and they were expecting not to be successful. Once the team had convinced themselves of the validity of requesting samples, they were able to put this across to respondents in a clear and persuasive manner. As it turned out that the majority of clubbers were providing samples each fieldwork night, interviewers' experience and confidence increased. Both the asking and the collecting of urine became another matter-of-fact, even mundane part of a busy and demanding fieldwork night.

We suspected that gender may have played a role in the success or failure of obtaining urine samples. We noted on the very first fieldwork night, for example:

We got seven urine samples, I think six men and one woman. I'm quite amazed at that really, even though it was only half of the planned 15. The first impression we got was the gendered nature of it. (1) the practicalities of not feeling able to easily get the urine into the pot. Technically, its easier for men to direct their aim, and also (2) culturally, men are more familiar with doing so, peeing in urinals, etc. Women are a bit more squeamish and embarrassed about urinating. I had thought this might be a problem from the start of our prolonged urine pot discussions, despite the assurances of the lab staff. It is difficult, particularly for the majority of clubbers who will have had drugs and alcohol and be a bit intoxicated. Some of the young teenage women at the club may never have given a sample in their lives and may just not know how to do it and not think it's possible. Also, women are going to think it's messy and be more put off than men about getting urine on their hands which is presumably a more regular occurrence for men! (3) On top of this is the dehydration issue. A couple of women took away pots and said that when they did go to the toilet later on, they'd do a sample and bring it back but they didn't. (Co-ordinator fieldwork notes)

In spite of our initial concerns, however, there were no significant differences between the proportion of female dance drug sample interviewees providing urine and male (60.2 per cent compared with 69.7 per cent). Whilst the gender of respondents did not appear to affect compliance rates in obtaining urine, the gender of research team members did play a role. Similar numbers of male respondents returned urine to both male and female fieldworkers. However, women were significantly less likely to return urine to our male fieldworkers.

Table 3.2   **Respondents returning urine to interviewers by gender**

	Male Interviewers	Female Interviewers	Both
Male respondents	68.4	70.6	69.7
Female respondents	47.7	73.0	60.2

What we don't know, beyond the anecdotal level, is the influence of the co-ordinators' gender (both of whom were female) on urine return rates. For some of the more reluctant respondents a more detailed discussion with the co-ordinators about the purpose behind the samples helped to sway them.

Craig's [male interviewer] woman dance drug respondent wouldn't do a urine sample so I had a word with her. Reassured her it's confidential, it's important research and we'd really appreciate it. She agreed. (Co-ordinator fieldwork notes)

We devised a number of strategies to deal with some of the practical problems in obtaining and storing urine in club surroundings. Firstly, urine specimen pots were issued in discreet brown bags, in which respondents then returned the filled pots. Returned pots were stored in a cool box. Prior to storage, pots were placed in labelled laboratory bags. This entailed handling of the pots, which we discovered were often not completely sealed, and therefore subject to spills. We dealt with this by placing instructions on the pot lids about how to seal them tightly, and additionally providing a verbal explanation to respondents. The research co-ordinator on each fieldwork night was responsible for the handling of the urine, and this was done wearing disposable gloves. Nevertheless, some pots were damaged in some way and leaks resulted.

> Table disaster! First someone knocked over Debbie's drink and it went all over the table and soaked Craig's leather jacket and various piles of paper. Then one of Debbie's full urine pots leaked a big puddle of piss over the table, which I mopped up, to all the team's disgust. Then I had to pour the rest into a new pot. Then I realised it had splashed my clipboard, so I mopped that up. (Co-ordinator fieldwork notes)

The limitations of in-club medical assessments

On reflection the pulse and temperature tests, although successfully undertaken, did not prove particularly effective at saying anything new about dancing on drugs. The physical environment in terms of varying temperatures, ever changing lighting conditions, both on the dance floor and as customers move around the venue, and the impossibility of control for exactly when a pulse is taken, all undermine the validity and reliability of the data. Our own view would be that such procedures may only be worth repeating in any future in-club studies with more sensitive equipment.

The veracity of the urinalysis is more complex and more heartening. Table 3.3 contains the percentage of respondents with a drug confirmed as present in their urine who also reported having consumed that drug on the fieldwork night by the time we interviewed them (i.e. 'true' positives). Respondents who self-reported consumption of amphetamine on the fieldwork night had the highest percentage (90 per cent) of positive urine tests for that drug. Ecstasy and cannabis followed at 60 per cent and 59 per cent and cannabis had the least correspondence at 48 per cent. These figures and particularly the highest figure for amphetamine go some way towards estimating the parameters of validity in self-reported use of illegal drugs in dance clubs. We suspect that the high correspondence between amphetamine self-report and urine tests was due in part to the fact that a disproportionate number of respondents tended to consume amphetamine prior to entry into the club (73 per cent of respondents ideally would take amphetamine prior to going to the club, compared to 44 per cent for ecstasy, 58 per cent for cannabis and 61 per cent for cocaine). This consumption pattern suggests that amphetamine would have had a longer period of time in order to 'show up' in urine. In fact, we knew during the fieldwork that some ecstasy users were providing urine samples within a relatively short period of time (an hour or less) of ingestion.

Table 3.3*   **Urine test results for dance drug sample**

Positive urine tests of respondents reporting drug use 'today'	
Amphetamine	90%
Ecstasy	60%
Cannabis	59%
Cocaine	48%
Positive urine tests of respondents not reporting drug use 'today'	
Amphetamine	22%
Cannabis	17%
Ecstasy	15%
Cocaine	2%

* base percentage is number of respondents self-reporting drug consumption.

The fact that the correspondence between urine tests and self-report data is lower for ecstasy, cannabis and cocaine than for amphetamines is interesting. Issues such as quality and purity of street drugs and the timing of consumption in relation to urination may in part explain these lower figures. For example, urine analyses revealed low levels of MDA (seven weak positives) in the urine of ecstasy users and given that MDA is a metabolite produced in the metabolising of ecstasy, this suggests that our urine samples were provided relatively soon after ecstasy consumption. Of course, these findings may suggest that club goers are more reluctant to reveal their use of ecstasy than amphetamines, perhaps relating to ecstasy being a Class A drug and amphetamines in non-injectable form being a Class B drug under the Misuse of Drugs Act. But this is unlikely because our respondents reported much 'serious' drug use, both past and present, in interviews and went to the trouble of volunteering urine samples.

The second part of the table also gauges validity of self-reported drug use in the club context, showing the numbers of respondents with positive urine tests who did not self-report use of the drug during the fieldwork day/evening. This occurred for about one in five or fewer respondents for each drug, although the discrepancy was highest for amphetamines (22 per cent).

We think the main reasons for this dissonance lie not in unreliable data from the interview or in the spiking of clubbers' drinks but in two other arenas. Firstly, our interviewees may have unwittingly consumed a drug because it was an adulterant in other drugs they had imbibed. This may particularly be the case with amphetamines, being a compound of what respondents believed to be an ecstasy tablet. Furthermore, amphetamine is a metabolite of ecstasy and may thus appear in the urine of people who did not purposefully take amphetamine. Secondly, the regularity of drug use amongst this sample and the fact that many were assessed late on Saturday night – the second partying night of the weekend for some – means we were probably identifying drug consumption which took place prior to the fieldwork period. On balance the urinanalysis results are consistent with the self-report data, the chronology of consumption and thus with accurate reporting by interviewees.

The evidence from the laboratory regarding the strength and purity of ecstasy consumed by our clubbers was mixed. On the one hand, we found that 24 dance drug users' samples tested positive for ketamine, although none of our dance drug users had indicated they had taken ketamine on the fieldwork night. This suggests that at the time of the fieldwork, ketamine was likely to have been sold as ecstasy. However, other evidence suggested that much of the ecstasy found in urine samples was strong. Of samples in which ecstasy was detected (88 of 221), it was 'strongly positive' in almost half of these (45.5 per cent). Furthermore, only 7 samples (3.2 per cent) were positive for MDA; 11 (5.0 per cent) were positive for ephedrine; and 1 (0.5 per cent) positive for MDEA, all found in tablets sold as 'ecstasy' in Britain. Although MDA is a metabolite of MDMA, the fact that this was only detected weakly in each case in which it was detected, suggests that when it showed it up in samples it was likely to have indeed been as a metabolite rather than having been directly orally consumed by clubbers. In fact, and in contrast to common perceptions of the quality of ecstasy illegally purchased in Britain in the late 1990s, the staff at the laboratory in which all the urine tests were carried out were surprised at the strength and purity of the MDMA found in the club samples and consequently had to raise the threshold of the measurement they categorise as 'strongly positive'.

If this device is to be reused in future club research the lessons are clear. The ideal setting is an 'all nighter' when drugs taken at the beginning to middle of the event have a better chance to be broken down and present in the urine. Alternatively, urine sampling should be undertaken as late as possible into the event for physiological if not for methodological reasons. It might also be pertinent to gather data on drug use across the previous seven days with great precision, including prescription drugs.

Representativeness of the samples

We have already acknowledged that there can be no veracious claims that our study provides a representative sample of dance clubs in general, let alone the broader night club sector. In this section we assess the representativeness of our sweep survey (N = 2,057) of the customer base of the three dance clubs and of the interviewees (n = 362) of the overall swept survey sample. We also consider the characteristics of the medical sub sample.

The overall club sample based on the sweep surveys was fairly evenly divided across the three clubs (see Table 3.3). Very roughly we undertook about a hundred sweeps per night in each club. However typical attendance at each club ranged from approximately 300–800 at the Warehouse club to 800–3,000 at the Leisure Centre and 500–800 at the City Centre club. Remembering we had a quota target of 1:1 by gender and 1:9 black/Asian to white respondents, perhaps a distorting factor, but that we made concerted attempts to evenly sweep customers soon after they entered the club, how likely is it that we obtained representativeness for the customer base?

Overall representativeness

We cannot unequivocally demonstrate that our survey samples are representative of the customer base but there are positive indications. Table 3.4 contains the sample characteristics, and shows that across all three clubs, with some variations, males, females, as well as black, white, and Asian respondents were represented. Numbers of black and Asian respondents, however, were still relatively few, so analyses in remaining chapters are not carried out by race. Nevertheless, the ethnic characteristics of our sample are roughly similar to that found in the population of the region in which the research was carried out (white – 94.1 per cent; black – 1.3 per cent; Asian – 4.0 per cent) (Census, 1991). Demographic characteristics of clubbers are discussed in further detail in Chapter 4.

Table 3.4   Sample characteristics

		Warehouse	*Leisure Centre*	*City Centre*	*Totals*
Club Sweep Sample		n = 707	n = 666	n = 684	N = 2057
Gender	Male	382 (54.0%)	368 (55.3%)	380 (55.6%)	1130 (54.9%)
	Female	325 (40.0%)	298 (44.7%)	304 (44.4%)	927 (45.1%)
Race	Black	31 (4.4%)	8 (1.2%)	17 (2.5%)	56 (2.7%)
	White	641 (90.0%)	650 (97.6%)	638 (93.3%)	1929 (93.9%)
	Asian	25 (3.5%)	4 (0.6%)	22 (3.2%)	51 (2.5%)

Also, we can see from Table 3.4 that the overall sample (N = 2,057) and samples within each of the clubs were large. Although we cannot make claims that samples on any one fieldwork night were representative of a club's customers since a random sampling technique could not be employed, these large sample sizes go some way to increasing the chances that our samples had some degree of representativeness of each club's customer base. One way that we can specifically address represenativeness, however, is through the analysis of non-responders; that is, those clubbers we approached for interview who refused.

Interviewers recorded details of their visual assessment of race and gender of those clubbers who were approached by the research team but refused to complete the initial brief sweep interview. In part these data allow us to determine in what ways those who refused to participate in the research differed from those who did participate, and whether or not, therefore, the resulting club sample (N = 2,057) was representative of club goers on the fieldwork nights.

We were also able to consider our refusal rate in relation to the race and gender of interviewers.

Of the recorded 2,191 clubbers we approached during the sweep surveys 134 (6.1 per cent) refused to participate. In respect of gender, a slightly higher proportion of women (6.6 per cent) than men (5.4 per cent) refused to complete sweep interviews but this difference was not statistically significant. Refusals were gendered, however, in the respect that both male and female respondents were more likely to decline a brief interview to male team members (7.5 per cent) than to females (4.5 per cent).

The race of both clubbers and researchers was significantly related to refusal rates. Black and Asian clubbers who were approached to complete the sweep interview were significantly more likely to refuse than white clubbers. Whilst only 5.1 per cent of white clubbers declined, 12.5 per cent of black clubbers and 21.5 per cent of Asian clubbers declined participation.

This disproportionate refusal rate is further illustrated when we look at the co-operation-refusal ratios for each of our fieldworkers. Our black fieldworker (British born of black African descent) had no refusals from black and Asian clubbers compared with a 15.3 per cent rate of these refusals for the remainder of the (white) team. Although our black fieldworker had an overall refusal rate lower than the norm, suggesting he was particularly effective at engaging clubbers anyway, this is all highly indicative. An impression of the team's 'whiteness' may well have played a part in discouraging black and Asian clubbers from participation.

This said, because we were operating on a 1:9 black/Asian:white quota during the sweep interviews this did not, in the end, wholly undermine our commitment to having ethnic minority representation. Just over 6 per cent of the survey sample were black or Asian, in line with the region's demographic profiles.

This race issue suggests that the trust process was important in distinguishing refusers from participants. Further evidence of this was found. In particular we found that refusal rates were higher in the first few nights of the fieldwork period at each club than on later nights when we had become established. At the City Centre club for instance the refusal rate on the first night was 9.2 per cent but dropped to 5.0 per cent on the second and 3.6 per cent on the third fieldwork night. Whilst there could be several reasons for this, our overall view is that the most potent factor was the initial suspicion/scepticism of clubbers about our appearance at 'their' club. However having talked with those clubbers who had co-operated on the first few fieldwork nights, seen no negative consequences of our enquiries over the weeks, had casual conversations with the research team and perhaps got used to our presence and wanderings, this suspicion tended to reduce:

Interestingly, I got a few reports from clubbers and from the research team about people beginning to trust us because of our continued presence. The two women I interviewed said that at the start they thought we were the police and were taking information to get people thrown out. She said that as the nights wore on they, and others, began to trust us more. (Co-ordinator fieldwork notes)

Refusal rates probably also dropped after the first night because of our use of posters distributed throughout the three fieldwork clubs. We designed colour posters explaining the purpose of the research project and assuring confidentiality to participants. The poster also explained:

This is the first large-scale independent study of the health of clubbers in the UK, conducted by professional researchers. We are not working for the police, or the management of this club.

At the beginning of the fieldwork night before staff opened the doors to customers, the research team pinned posters on all available wall surfaces; around the reception area, on the walls inside the club, at appropriate locations for customers to read such as near cigarette machines, near queues for the bar and toilets, and on all toilet cubicle doors, inside and out. The posters proved to be a talking-point and were read by almost everyone in the club. They helped to explain our presence to those people we didn't speak to, provided extra details about the research project and helped to reassure those who had doubts about our identity. In subsequent weeks, customers would engage in conversation with us having read the posters, sometimes agreeing to interviews they had previously refused, having been 'won over' during the course of our presence over several weeks in each of the three clubs.

Refusal rates also differed significantly by individual interviewer, and ranged from 1.2 per cent to 11.4 per cent. There are a number of potential reasons for the variation in refusal rates. Firstly, and most obviously, it may be that some interviewers were simply better or more persuasive at obtaining the consent of club goers to participate. However, it is likely that other explanations were also at work. As discussed earlier, team members were instructed to approach clubbers to a gender ratio of 1:1, and to a race ratio of 9:1 white:black/Asian. We have already seen that the gender and race of interviewers affected their 'success' rates in obtaining sweep interviews, and it is likely therefore that other interviewer characteristics also affected refusal rates. Secondly, therefore, respondents may have been influenced by interviewer characteristics in deciding whether to agree to be interviewed, an interview that was, after all, visible to other clubbers, indeed a 'display' in the public and image-conscious context of the club. A whole series of interviewer characteristics may have been at work here: age or 'youthfulness', 'trendyness', perceived attractiveness, friendliness, availability and so on. Thirdly, as discussed above in relation to race and gender, is the unconscious bias of interviewers in selecting respondents. So, for example, interviewers may have consciously or unconsciously attempted to 'target' clubbers who appeared to them to be amenable to participation in the research, who appeared approachable, or who appeared attractive or interesting. Fourthly, it is possible that some team members failed to record refusals as such. This may not have been a deliberate attempt at deception, although particularly early on in their employment on the project, refusals may have been seen by research team members as them failing to do their jobs properly and therefore something they may not wish to make record of. The research co-ordinators were very keen to collect data on refusals, and therefore clarified definitions of refusals in our weekly fieldwork updates and reassured team members that it was for research purposes rather than managerial purposes that we were interested in individual refusal rates.

The interview sample compared to the club sample who were not interviewed

Of the 2,057 sweep interviews that comprised the club sample, 362 (16.5 per cent) were interviewed. In order to determine how representative the interview sample was of the club sample, comparisons were made between the 362 members of the club sample who were interviewed and the 1,695 who were not.

There were no significant differences between the two samples in relation to gender, employment status, class, race, sexual orientation, and club in which the research was carried out. The interview sample, however, was significantly older (mean = 23.9 years) than the club sample who were not interviewed (mean = 22.6 years), although the difference was small at only 1.4 years ($p < 0.001$). There were also small differences by social class ($p < 0.05$). The interview sample had somewhat more respondents in the managerial/professional class (27.0 per cent) than the club sample not interviewed (22.8 per cent); as well, the interview sample had somewhat fewer students (22.1 per cent compared to 30.0 per cent).

There were no significant differences between the samples in terms of whether respondents drank alcohol, frequency of alcohol consumption, and tobacco smoking. However, the interview sample had considerably more drug involvement. In particular, they were more likely to have taken or be planning to take a drug on the fieldwork night (89.0 per cent compared to 59.6 per cent) ($p < 0.001$). Their past three month usage of at least one drug was also somewhat higher (93.6 per cent compared to 81.9 per cent) ($p < 0.001$). This suggests that they were likely to have been more frequent or regular drug users.

We were also interested in the extent to which respondents who agreed to an interview may have done so in part due to the effects of drugs already taken, and in particular suspected that the effects of ecstasy may have made respondents more amenable to us. Here we compared all those having been asked for an interview (N = 765) who subsequently agreed to be interviewed (n = 471, 61.6 per cent) (whether or not they actually had been interviewed), to those who refused an interview (n = 294, 38.4 per cent). Contrary to our expectation, but reassuringly, those who agreed to an interview were no more likely than those who refused to have already consumed ecstasy when we asked them. The same was true for amphetamines, cannabis and cocaine. Although there were no differences between these two groups in numbers who had already consumed alcohol, however, those agreeing to an interview had consumed significantly more alcohol (mean of 8.3 units) compared to those who refused (6.6 units, $p < 0.01$).

In summary, we can conclude that the interview sample was not substantially different from the club sample in terms of demographic characteristics and their consumption of alcohol and tobacco. However, the interview sample is likely to have contained more regular drug users. Contrary to expectation, however, those agreeing to an interview were no more likely to have taken ecstasy or other illicit drugs than those refusing an interview, although they had consumed significantly more alcohol.

This is an important finding. Our worries that the effects of ecstasy in particular may have made potential research participants more compliant may have been unfounded. However, the effects of intoxication by poly drug use and/or alcohol may well have played a role in compliance.

The dance drug interviewees compared to the medical sub sample

Of the interview dance drug sample (N = 317), 54 respondents (17.0 per cent) attended for an in-depth medical assessment. In order to determine the representativeness of the medical sub sample, they were compared to those not in the sub sample (n = 263).

There were no significant differences between the two samples in relation to gender, employment status, class, race, sexual orientation, and club in which the research was carried out. The medical sub sample, however, was significantly ($p < .0.05$) older (mean = 25.7 years) than those not in the sub sample (mean = 23.7 years), a difference of two years.

There were no differences between the two samples in terms of whether respondents drank alcohol, drinking frequency and smoking tobacco. There were also no differences in whether respondents in each sample considered themselves to be users of speed, cannabis, ecstasy, or cocaine. There were no differences either in total amounts of these drugs consumed on the fieldwork night or in typical amounts consumed. Members of the medical sub sample were slightly more frequent users of ecstasy (mean of 55.8 times per year) than those not in the sub sample (39.9 times per year) ($p < 0.05$). There were no differences in frequency of use for the other drugs, however.

Again, this suggests that the medical sub sample was remarkably similar to the dance drug-using interview sample, in spite of the fact that this group was a self-selecting volunteer sample.

Conclusion

Undertaking research inside functioning dance clubs and night clubs is clearly feasible (see also Release, 1997; Newcombe, 1992a). There will be some venues where the conditions, particularly too much noise and too little personal space, would restrict research activities but certainly in larger clubs it is possible to find quieter areas and appropriate places to site the fieldwork base.

There is a trade-off however in terms of applying 'scientific' research procedures. We have described how difficult it was to sample club entrants and to find clubbers we were monitoring in packed venues. Hearing every word a respondent utters is difficult, privacy during the interview cannot be guaranteed and taping is infeasible. On the other hand, none of our procedures were undermined or invalidated by working in busy clubs, there was no sense that the usual techniques didn't work, that sampling was ineffective or that respondents, despite their primary goal of enjoying their night out, were untruthful or dismissive. Those that participated did so purposefully and enthusiastically for the most part, so that aside from the small refusal rate at the sweep stage and the intoxication issue in relation to interviewing people in their leisure settings, we were able to conduct high-quality interviews and assessments. We would suggest, therefore, that flexibility and reflexivity rather than standardisation and uniformity are preferable methodological approaches to research in night-time leisure settings.

We were, however, always apprehensive and thus alert to the potential for things to go wrong and this was our stimulant drug to ensure nothing was left to chance. The elaborate protocols, training, health and safety measures, on-going adaptations and constant commitment to fine detail almost certainly prevented a number of unwanted situations developing. This said, there is little doubt we were also 'lucky' because some contingencies cannot be planned for or overcome. There are assaults, fights, there is always someone looking for trouble, the police do raid venues, people do get sexually assaulted. We witnessed all of these events but luckily never got disproportionately involved in them. However there is no doubt that even the most professional and well-organised project could get caught up in trouble or upset. It would be unwise to undertake club fieldwork with any sense of invulnerability.

The paucity of empirical research in such a key social environment as clubland is perhaps a product of this perceived 'dangerousness', combined with the demise in both funding and commitment to naturalistic fieldwork in the social sciences. The end result is that what are enormous difficulties in achieving representativeness are compounded by a lack of research replication and elaboration. We have undertaken the largest independent academic study of UK dance drug use in clubs so far and yet can make no supportable claims of representativeness beyond the customers of the three clubs we investigated.

We can now begin to present the findings of this study. The sweep and interview samples form the basis of the next chapter in which we look at who the clubbers are, what drugs they take and where, when and how often. Chapter 5 relies primarily on the interview samples, the in-club monitoring and some results from the medical assessments. In Chapter 6 we utilise the interview samples' data, our observations and informal interviews with 'professionals' and club staff to describe and discuss issues relating to violence, safety and security in clubland.

4 The Clubbers and their Nights Out

In this chapter we look in detail at who the clubbers are and what they do on their nights out. The analysis is based on the sweep survey of over 2,000 dance club customers and the detailed interviews with, primarily, over 300 regular dance drug users. We begin by describing who the clubbers are in terms of gender, age, ethnicity, sexual orientation and socio-economic status. We then describe their alcohol, tobacco and illicit drug antecedents before looking at their recent and current use of psycho-active substances.

This all helps us understand how the clubbers have become such committed and regular poly drug users whereby on their nights out in clubland, we find a clear strategy for maximising their enjoyment of a long night. Their choice of drugs, including alcohol, the dosage, the timing and order of administration are all part of their purposeful approach.

Who are the clubbers?

Table 4.1 contains the demographic characteristics of the full club sample (N = 2,057). The somewhat higher proportion of males (54.9 per cent), despite an attempted gender quota of 1:1 employed in the sweep survey, reflects the disproportionate numbers of males in these venues. This over-representation of males in clubs is also reflected in other surveys (e.g., McElrath and McEvoy, 1999; Release, 1997), though it is not universal (Handy et al., 1998). The club sample was also predominantly white (93.9 per cent), again reflecting the under-representation of non-whites in the chosen clubs, in spite of the attempted quota sampling strategy of 9:1 white:black/Asian respondents. Although other surveys have also suggested an over-representation of white clubgoers (e.g., Release 1997), the proportion of black and Asian respondents found is similar to their proportion in population figures for the region (see Chapter 3). However, as Table 4.1 also shows, ethnicity did significantly vary by club (p < .001), with, in particular, the Leisure Centre having a higher percentage of white customers (97.6 per cent) than the other two clubs in this study.

These differences in customer base between just three different mainstream dance clubs is a clear illustration of the diversity of clubs and their relative attractiveness to different clubbers. It reinforces the point we made in the last chapter about the practical impossibility of achieving representativeness in club research.

We reach the same conclusion when we consider sexual orientation. Whilst we purposefully chose one club with a gay/lesbian customer profile, the differences are stark. Whilst more than three-quarters (76.6 per cent) of the sweep survey sample identified themselves as 'straight' or heterosexual, compared to 17.8 per cent who were gay/lesbian and 5.7 per cent who were bisexual, the vast majority of gay/lesbian (98.4 per cent) and bisexual (76.7 per cent) club goers were found in the City Centre club.

Table 4.1   Demographic characteristics of the club sample

N = 2057	Total		Warehouse	Leisure Centre	City Centre
	n	%	%	%	%
Male	1130	54.9	54.0	55.3	55.6
Female	927	45.1	46.0	44.7	44.4
White	1929	93.9	90.9	97.6	93.3
Black	56	2.7	4.4	1.2	2.5
Asian	51	2.5	3.5	0.6	3.2
Other	19	0.9	1.1	0.6	1.0
Straight	1572	76.6	96.3	98.9	34.4
Gay/lesbian	365	17.8	0.9	0.0	52.6
Bisexual	116	5.7	2.8	1.1	13.0
Age					
15–17	49	2.4	1.3	5.0	1.0
18–20	845	41.3	39.9	57.1	27.5
21–25	660	32.3	36.2	28.5	31.9
26–30	321	15.7	16.8	6.1	23.9
31–57	170	8.3	5.8	3.3	15.7
Age (mean)	2045	22.8 years	22.7 years	20.7 years	24.9 years

Missing data: ethnicity (2); sexual orientation (4); age (12).

The age of the club sample ranged from 15 to 57 with a mean of 22.8 years (s.d. = 5.06). The largest proportion of respondents were in the age range from 18 to 20 years, and the majority of club goers overall (73.6 per cent) in the club sample were in their late teens and early twenties. A very small minority (2.4 per cent) were under the legal age for the purchase of alcoholic drinks (18 years) in the venues in which our research took place. A significant minority (8.3 per cent) were over the age of 30. The age distribution was fairly similar to that found in the other surveys (Akram, 1997; Release, 1997). The City Centre club had the highest proportion of over thirties (15.7 per cent compared to under 6 per cent in the other two clubs) whereas the Leisure Centre had the highest proportion of younger customers and those underage for the purchase of alcoholic drinks. The average age was highest in the City Centre club (24.9 years) and lowest in the Leisure Centre (20.7 years). Age is thus one more factor in self-selection by customers although this is also shaped by door policies at individual clubs.

Table 4.2 contains the frequency distributions for employment status and socio-economic class[1] for the club sample. The key finding here is that clubbers came from a wide range of socio-economic backgrounds. The vast majority of club goers in the club sample – over eight in ten – were either employed full-time (58.4 per cent) or in higher education (24.4 per cent). Only about 1 in 20 were unemployed. This suggests that clubbers appear to be predominantly economically active and contributing to the mainstream economy, rather than dislocated from participation in productive employment or training. This finding is consistent with other studies which also suggest that clubbers come from all social backgrounds. For those who were working, their occupations were coded into three social class groupings. This also suggests a profile of clubbers that in no way reflects marginalisation: nearly a quarter (23.5 per cent) were in the managerial or professional job classifications, and 15.4 per cent were employed in jobs classed as intermediate. About one-third were in the 'working' job classification: primarily manual along with routine services. Most other studies have noted this diversity although some have found a small minority from the grey or criminal economy (Hammersley et al., 1999; McElrath and McEvoy, 1999) not identified in our brief sweep survey.

Table 4.2   Employment status and socio-economic class of the club sample

N = 2057	Total		Warehouse	Leisure Centre	City Centre
	n	%	%	%	%
Employment status					
Full-time employed	1190	58.4	51.9	65.3	58.6
Higher education	497	24.4	37.9	4.9	29.5
Unemployed	111	5.4	2.7	9.6	4.3
Further education	87	4.3	3.0	8.5	1.5
Part-time employed	87	4.3	–	–	–
Carer	32	1.6	–	–	–
Job training	14	0.7	–	–	–
Sick/disabled	14	0.7	–	–	–
School	3	0.1	–	–	–
Other	2	0.1	–	–	–
SE class					
Managerial and professional	472	23.6	26.1	13.3	30.5
Intermediate	308	15.4	13.5	16.8	16.0
Working	650	32.4	19.3	56.3	23.7
Students	574	28.6	41.1	13.6	29.8

Missing data: employment status (20); SE class (630) including unclassifiable occupations

The three clubs did vary in terms of the socio-economic profile of their customers however, and these differences were statistically significant (p < 0.001). The Leisure Centre, although having the highest proportion of respondents in full-time employment (65.3 per cent) had the fewest customers in the professional/managerial category, the fewest students, the highest proportion in the routine and manual occupations, and the highest proportion of customers who were unemployed. The City Centre club had the largest proportion of respondents in the highest grouping, and the Warehouse club had the most students. This suggests that music policy, location, club atmosphere and door policy are likely to affect the kind of clientele a club attracts; however, consistent with other research, all three clubs attracted a varied customer base reflecting a range of socio-economic backgrounds, with a probable over-representation of the managerial/professional group, particularly if we accept that higher education students tend to find eventual employment in this sector.

In short, the beginning point for any discussion about clubs and dance drugs in the UK must be with the demographic characteristics of the customer base. Young clubbers are in these terms ordinary, normative and representative of their age cohort. There were very few differences in demographic characteristics between those who were and were not recent dance drug users. They cannot, therefore, be pathologised or theorised to the social or economic margins where this status is then intuitively linked with illegal drug use.

Clubbers as psycho-active consumers

Heavy smokers and drinkers

The alcohol and tobacco profiles of the overall club sample (see Table 4.3) suggest that dance club goers have substantially higher use of these substances than the

Table 4.3   Alcohol and tobacco use in the club sample (N = 2057)

N = 2057	n	%
Drinking status:		
Current drinker	1978	96.2
Stopped drinking	57	2.8
Never drank alcohol	22	1.1
Drinking frequency:		
<1 weekly	183	9.3
once weekly	313	15.9
2–3 weekly	820	41.7
most/all days weekly	651	33.1
Current smoker	1401	68.1
Ex-smoker	201	9.8
Daily smoker	1157	82.6

rest of the population. All but a handful were current drinkers, and most (74.8 per cent) drank more than once a week. About one-third (33.1 per cent) estimated that they drank most or all days of the week. Whilst 18- to 24-year-olds and especially males are the heaviest drinkers in the population these rates correspond with the most alcohol involved for the age group (Wright, 1999). Current tobacco smoking (68.1 per cent) is over twice the rate for the general population (ONS, 1998). Furthermore, given that most smokers were daily smokers (82.6 per cent), this suggests that the club is not simply a setting where those who are generally non-smokers just occasionally indulge.

Lifetime and recent drug-taking experience

The key conclusion to be drawn from Table 4.4 is that clubbers are extremely drug-experienced. The vast majority (94.1 per cent) have ever tried a drug compared with around half (49 per cent for the 16–19 age group, 55 per cent for 20- to 24-year-olds) identified in household surveys (Ramsay and Partridge, 1999). The lifetime rates for the specific listed drugs are also far higher than found in household or school and college surveys. For example, we find lifetime drug experience amongst 11- to 35-year-olds in England for amphetamines at around 16 per cent ever used and with ecstasy 7 per cent ever used (HEA, 1999). These rates are far lower than those found amongst the clubbers.

Table 4.4   Lifetime and past three month prevalence figures for selected drugs in the club sample (N = 2057)

Drug	Lifetime	Past 3 months
Cannabis	86.8	69.5
Speed	76.8	53.5
Poppers	71.9	30.0
Ecstasy	67.3	51.4
LSD	52.0	14.6
Cocaine powder	44.9	27.1
Legal herbal drugs	38.0	17.8
Tranquillisers	15.4	6.3
GHB	10.6	5.5
Crack	7.0	2.4
Heroin	6.0	1.6
Viagra	2.9	1.7
At least one	94.1	84.0

The only other drug-using group with these levels of lifetime experience and high rates of recent use[2] are 'problem' drug users who are 'career' heroin, crack cocaine users (e.g. Brain et al., 1998; Power, 1995). However, as we shall see, this is where close similarities end.

We can also identify from Table 4.4 that cannabis is the most-used illicit drug. Although the rate of recent use is far higher than in the general young adult population, it parallels the significance of the drug in the wider population. There are also clues in this table about the sample's approach to drug use. They have embraced cocaine far more than their predecessors from the early 1990s and have a clear tendency to try 'new' drugs even with problematic reputations. GHB (gamma hydroxy butyrate) in particular only became easily available at the end of the 1990s, yet we find over one in ten of the sweep interviewees having already tried it. Similarly, we found that supplies of newly licensed Viagra became quickly available on the club scene during our fieldwork in the final club in the autumn of 1998. We immediately revised the sweep schedule and managed to ask 519 respondents about Viagra and consequently generated a 2.9 per cent trying rate in the City Centre club. This willingness to try new drugs despite stepping into the unknown fundamentally distinguishes the clubbers from the far more cautious risk assessments and drug taking of their age peers as described in Chapter 1. On the other hand, our clubbers largely continue to eschew crack cocaine and heroin, thereby distinguishing themselves from, as they see it, dependent drug users.

The dance drug users and non-users distinguished

We can sophisticate the clubbers' profile by distinguishing between those who were using dance drugs on the fieldwork night (the 'users' – 1,057, or 51.4 per cent of the club sample) from those who were not (the 'non-users') in respect of their alcohol, tobacco and illicit drug statuses. Table 4.5 suggests that there are only small differences in respect of smoking and drinking. Both sub samples appear to be regular current drinkers who drink with roughly similar frequency. Their alcohol consumption over the course of the night was somewhat higher, but this is not surprising given that they were not combining their alcohol use with stimulant-based drug use. Non-dance drug users are still far more likely to smoke than their age group in the general population, but are somewhat less likely to be current smokers than their dance drug-using peers.

Turning to illicit drug use, the differences are, as expected, far more substantial (see Table 4.6). The dance drug users were significantly more likely to have more lifetime drug experience of all drugs (except Viagra and legal herbal drugs). This said, the non-users, as clubbers, are still very experienced. They may not be current dance drug users, but most have at least tried these drugs and again at rates which distinguish them from the general younger population.

In summary, whilst the current dance drug sweep interviewees are very drug-experienced, even clubbers who had not used a dance drug for two years were still exceptionally drug-experienced.

Table 4.5   Alcohol and tobacco use of dance drug users v. non-dance drug users in the club sample (N = 2057)

	Total (N = 2057)	Non-Users (n = 1000)	Users (n = 1057)	Sig
Drinking status:				
Current drinker	96.2	96.8	95.6	}ns
Stopped drinking	2.8	2.0	3.5	
Never drank alcohol	1.1	1.2	0.9	
Drinking frequency:				
<1 weekly	9.3	6.7	11.8	}ns
once weekly	15.9	16.4	15.5	
2–3 weekly	41.7	47.3	36.3	
most/all days weekly	33.1	29.6	36.4	
Mean alcohol:				
units consumed	7.83	8.03	7.63	ns
units planned	6.13	6.26	5.93	ns
total	9.59	11.05	8.19	***
Current smoker	68.1	59.7	76.1	}***
Ex-smoker	9.8	12.6	7.1	
Daily smoker	82.6	77.4	86.6	***

Table 4.6   Lifetime prevalence of selected drugs of dance drug users v. non-dance drug users (N = 2057)

	Total (N = 2057)	Non-Users (n = 1000)	Users (n = 1057)	Sig
Cannabis	86.8	77.5	95.6	***
Speed	76.8	55.6	97.0	***
Poppers	71.9	57.4	85.5	***
Ecstasy	67.3	43.8	89.5	***
Legal herbal drugs	62.0	65.8	58.5	***
LSD	52.0	31.0	71.9	***
Cocaine powder	44.9	27.1	61.7	***
Tranquillisers	15.4	7.3	23.1	***
GHB	10.6	5.2	15.7	***
Crack	7.0	3.5	10.3	***
Heroin	6.0	3.1	8.7	***
Viagra	2.9	3.3	2.4	ns
At least one	94.1	87.9	100.0	***

Table 4.7   Lifetime and past three month prevalence of selected drugs for interview dance drug sample v. comparison sample (N = 362)

	Users (n = 317)	Comparison (n = 45)	Sig
Lifetime:			
Cannabis	96.2	68.9	***
Speed	96.8	37.8	***
Poppers	87.7	48.9	***
Ecstasy	95.3	35.6	***
Legal herbal drugs	42.6	36.6	ns
LSD	75.6	18.2	***
Cocaine powder	66.2	17.8	***
Tranquillisers	24.9	2.2	***
GHB	16.8	2.2	**
Crack	10.8	4.4	ns
Heroin	7.6	2.2	ns
Viagra	1.1	0.0	ns
At least one	100.0	80.8	***
Past three months:			
Cannabis	87.7	31.1	***
Speed	78.5	–	–
Poppers	42.0	15.6	***
Ecstasy	87.1	–	–
Legal herbal drugs	17.0	6.7	ns
LSD	23.7	–	–
Cocaine powder	42.9	–	–
Tranquillisers	11.0	0.0	*
GHB	9.5	0.0	*
Crack	3.5	–	–
Heroin	2.8	0.0	ns
Viagra	0.0	0.0	–
At least one	100.0	48.9	***

Drugs careers of interview sample

Turning now to the interview sample (N = 362) made up of the dance drug users (n = 317) and the comparison group (n = 45), we offer a more detailed profile of today's clubbers. Remembering that the comparison sample have not taken a key dance drug for at least two years, the overall impression from Table 4.7 is still of extensive drug use. Lifetime rates of dance drug use are four to nine times higher than in the wider same-age population as measured by household interviews. Even compared with higher education students (Pirie and Worcester, 1999; Webb et al., 1996) these rates are still far greater. On the other hand there is an absence of recent drug use (beyond cannabis) compared with the dance drug interviewees.

We specifically asked all the interviewees whether they considered themselves to be *users* of the listed drugs. This self-definition is revealing, showing that only five drugs – cannabis (51.7 per cent), amphetamines (36.8 per cent), ecstasy (46.0 per cent), cocaine powder (10.3 per cent) and amyl nitrite (9.2 per cent) – attracted significant self-nomination. Taking a drug ever or occasionally is not necessarily the same as defining oneself as a user. This self-definition of user further reminds us that past month consumption is a poor proxy for measuring current regular drug use (see Aldridge et al., 1999) tending, nearly always, to over-estimate. We can too easily allow traditional recency measures like 'past three month' therefore to over-alarm. Thus concerns across Europe about ketamine or GHB based on lifetime and recency measures would find further fuel in the rates in Table 4.8. Yet it becomes clear that they are primarily measuring experimentation or trying levels rather than scale of use or regular usage when we assess self-definitions of user status. Whilst trying some of these drugs does carry dangers, the point clubbers have made to us is that they learn from their experimentation and step back from becoming users of 'problematic' substances.

Table 4.8   Drugs history for interview sample (N=362): lifetime, past year and 'users' (%)

Drug	Lifetime (%)	Past month (%)	Self-defined user (%)	Yearly frequency* (mean)
Cannabis	93.1	74.0	51.7	261
Amphetamines	91.7	65.4	36.8	56
Ecstasy	87.7	69.6	46.0	43
Poppers	85.8	29.5	9.2	80
LSD	70.1	10.2	3.9	66
Cocaine powder	62.4	31.2	10.3	52
Mushrooms (dried)	41.9	3.7	2.2	–
Mushrooms (fresh)	40.1	2.8	2.2	–
Legal herbal drugs	33.6	5.6	2.5	–
Solvents	27.7	0.8	0.0	–
Tranquillisers	25.3	7.6	2.0	–
Ketamine	23.3	2.8	0.6	–
GHB	15.4	3.1	0.3	–
Crack cocaine	9.0	1.7	0.6	–
Opium	7.3	0.0	0.0	–
Heroin	6.7	1.1	0.6	–
Barbiturates	5.9	0.3	0.0	–
Methadone	5.3	0.6	0.0	–
Steroids	2.5	0.0	0.0	–
Viagra	0.6	0.3	0.0	–
At least one	97.8	92.5	76.5	–

– denotes too few cases (< 10) for meaningful analysis
*based on those who nominated themselves as users of these drugs

Gender, age, and club differences in drugs consumption

Given the exceptionally high rates of multiple drug experience amongst the club survey sample, it is worth exploring the impact of age, gender and club of choice. Whilst the gender differences in rates of drug trying have narrowed across the last decade and have almost disappeared amongst adolescents, we still find more male than female involvement in adulthood and with problematic drugs careers.

This picture is reinforced by the sweep survey results. We can see from Table 4.9 statistically significant gender differences run through the main illicit drugs. It is only at the margins with legal herbal drugs, crack and Viagra that differences are absent. However, the gendered distinctions of drug use should not overshadow the key finding that both female and male clubbers are remarkably drug-experienced.

Table 4.10 provides further detail to our understanding of how setting or club of choice affects rates of particular drugs consumption. Each of our clubs as commercial operations aim for a particular market segment and indeed through-door policy can exclude certain potential customers. We have already described the consequences of this on the customer base. But equally, potential clubbers will also, within these constraints, make choices about where to spend their nights out. These factors are reflected in the results in Table 4.10. The younger, more working-class, hardcore 'rave' crowd at the Leisure Centre are most likely to regard amphetamines and ecstasy as their dance drugs of choice and to have

Table 4.9   Lifetime prevalence rates by gender and age for the club survey sample (N = 2057)

Drug	M	F	sig	15–17	18–20	21–25	26–30	31–57	sig
Cannabis	88.6	84.6	**	81.6	88.5	86.5	84.1	86.5	ns
Amphetamines	79.6	73.5	**	73.5	74.3	80.8	75.6	78.2	*
Poppers	76.4	66.3	***	63.3	66.6	75.9	75.6	78.2	***
Ecstasy	73.1	60.2	***	53.1	58.9	73.8	73.4	77.1	***
LSD	56.6	46.5	***	44.9	46.8	57.6	50.8	59.4	***
Cocaine powder	51.1	37.3	***	24.5	34.7	50.9	55.1	60.4	***
Legal herbal drugs	39.4	36.2		16.3	38.6	39.8	40.3	29.4	**
Tranquillisers	18.2	12.0	***	14.3	12.9	15.9	18.8	19.4	ns
GHB	14.5	5.8	***	2.0	5.8	11.8	16.6	20.6	***
Crack	8.2	5.4	*	6.1	5.5	6.4	10.7	9.5	*
Heroin	7.8	3.8	***	2.0	2.7	7.3	10.3	10.0	***
Viagra (n = 519)	3.4	2.2	ns	0.0	1.7	3.6	2.3	4.1	ns
At least one (not including alcohol)	95.3	92.0	***	89.8	94.1	94.4	93.1	96.6	ns

* p < 0.05; ** p < 0.01; *** p < 0.001

less access to more expensive cocaine powder. With the City Centre club having the oldest and most affluent customer base we are unsurprised at their particularly extensive drug experience, for instance in respect of cocaine powder and GHB. Once again, however, we can see how age does not correlate with drug experience in a uni-linear fashion. The Leisure Centre has the youngest customer base yet in terms of lifetime trying of illicit drugs overall, the highest rate.

Table 4.10   Lifetime prevalence rates by club venue (N = 2057)

Drug	Warehouse	Leisure Centre	City Centre	sig
Cannabis	85.9	90.8	83.7	***
Amphetamines	72.4	86.0	72.5	***
Poppers	66.9	72.5	76.4	***
Ecstasy	66.1	71.0	65.0	*
LSD	48.9	62.5	45.1	***
Cocaine powder	46.3	37.7	50.4	***
Legal herbal drugs	41.2	33.5	39.0	*
Tranquillisers	13.9	17.0	15.4	ns
GHB	6.9	4.4	20.5	***
Crack	6.8	6.2	7.8	ns
Heroin	6.6	3.8	7.5	**
Viagra (n = 519)	–	–	2.9	ns
At least one (not including alcohol)	92.2	95.8	94.4	*

* p < 0.05; ** p < 0.01; *** p < 0.001

Very young clubbers as dance drug users

Returning to Table 4.9, we can see differences in lifetime prevalence rates for specific drugs between the age bands groups and that the over-thirties group is demonstrated to be the most drug-experienced. The remarkable feature, however, is just how small the differences are overall. The 15- to 20-year-old clubbers appear to have gained quite exceptional rates of drug experience in a very brief period during their adolescence.

The pace at which the youngest, teenage clubbers have accumulated illicit drug experience is one of the most significant findings in the sweep survey analysis. This is confirmed by looking at age of initiation into drug use by age group (Table 4.11). Here we find evidence that the drugs pathways from early adolescent drug trying into early clubbing and related recreational drug use cover only a few years. Today's young clubbers, the children of the 1990s, have tried a whole range of drugs, and in a recognisable order, several years earlier than their club elders. We also found that age was unrelated to either frequency of use or quantity of use (both on the fieldwork night and on an ideal night) for amphetamines, cannabis, ecstasy and cocaine (one exception to this was a positive correlation (Pearson's r = 0.376, p < 0.05, n = 36) between frequency of cocaine use and age such that older cocaine users consumed cocaine more often than younger users, although this was based on only a small number of users (n = 36) for whom data were available). Thus, younger dance drug users appear to be consuming similar drugs in similar quantities and roughly as often as their older counterparts. All this fits consistently with the normalisation of adolescent recreational drug use across the 1990s and the fall in the age of initiation across the board (McKeganey and Norrie, 1999; Aldridge et al., 1999). And finally when we look at how gender relates to age of initiation we find, for the overall interview sample, that females initiated slightly earlier than males for most of the key drugs (e.g. amphetamines (n = 327), males at 18.4 years, females at 18.0 years; ecstasy (n = 312), males at 19.8 years, females at 17.4 years).

Table 4.11   Mean age of initiation for interview sample (N = 362) by age group

Drug	15–17	18–20	21–25	26–30	31+
Solvents (n=98)	–	13.41	14.50	13.73	15.73
Cannabis (n=334)	13.14	14.06	15.43	16.72	21.45
LSD (n=247)	11.25	15.31	16.71	19.07	22.59
Mushrooms (fresh) (n=141)	–	15.24	16.92	18.38	22.57
Mushrooms (dried) (n=146)	–	15.59	17.16	18.31	22.96
Poppers (n=304)	11.40	15.39	16.92	19.62	25.79
Amphetamines (n=327)	12.20	15.75	17.10	20.41	24.56
Methadone (n=19)	–	–	18.88	20.67	–
Heroin (n=23)	–	–	19.73	21.17	–
Tranquillisers (n=83)	–	15.97	18.81	22.54	27.89
Ecstasy (n=312)	12.80	16.44	18.00	21.59	28.76
Barbiturates (n=21)	–	–	18.89	21.40	–
Opium (n=26)	–	–	20.25	18.80	23.40
Legal herbal drugs (n=116)	–	16.66	19.41	22.20	30.27
Ketamine (n=67)	–	17.26	19.24	21.67	29.56
Crack cocaine (n=31)	–	18.10	20.00	24.60	–
Cocaine powder (n=222)	–	17.67	20.31	23.77	27.79
GHB (n=54)	–	18.21	21.67	26.00	33.91
Steroids (n=9)	–	–	–	–	–
Viagra (n=1)	–	–	–	–	–

– indicates fewer than 5 respondents in age band

The clubbers' night out

In this section we describe the alcohol and drugs consumption patterns typically associated with a night out clubbing. Remembering the 'time out' context we have described in earlier chapters, we look here at the typical nature and timing of psycho-active consumption for club goers in our three venues. The basic ingredients of alcohol, cannabis, amphetamines, ecstasy and cocaine are mixed in a variety of ways. This poly drug approach, whilst evolving with fashion into the new millennium, is consistent with the other UK dance drug studies.

Drinking rates and roles

Table 4.12 describes the extent of alcohol consumption on the fieldwork night. Over three-quarters (78.2 per cent) of the club sample had already consumed alcohol by the time of the sweep interview, when clubbers had recently arrived, thereby confirming that the night out often began with drinking at home or in bars and pubs. By this time, on average, clubbers had consumed 7.83 units[3] of alcohol. Almost two-thirds of the clubbers (63.7 per cent) anticipated beginning or extending alcohol consumption across the night, and estimated on average consuming 6.13 units. The majority of the sample, therefore (83.6 per cent) either had already consumed alcohol or anticipated doing so, and average estimates for consumption over the course of the whole evening were 11.51 units in total. This suggests that many clubbers were drinking alcohol to the point of intoxication.

Table 4.12   Alcohol and drugs in combination (N = 2057)

N = 2057	% any	mean
Mean alcohol:		
units consumed	78.2	7.83
units planned	63.7	6.13
Total	83.6	11.51
Consumption plans for evening:	n	%
Mainly/only drinking	906	45.3
Mainly/only drugs	531	24.2
Both drinking & drugs	470	23.5
Neither drinking nor drugs	93	4.7

These figures indicate that alcohol is the key psycho-active substance consumed by nearly all clubbers. In fact, just under half (45.3 per cent) considered themselves to be mainly or only drinking on the fieldwork night. Combined with the roughly one in four (23.5 per cent) clubbers who considered themselves to be drinking and drug taking in equal measures, we can see that the vast majority (68.8 per cent) identified alcohol as a key part of the psycho-active mix. Most clubbers, perhaps unlike in the early acid house and 'rave' scene (see Chapter 2), appear to be taking alcohol and drugs together. The mixing of alcohol and dance drugs found in this study echoes the findings of other 1990s studies (e.g. Hammersley et al., 1999; Release, 1997).

Table 4.13 illustrates the variation in alcohol consumption by club. Customers at the Leisure Centre were significantly less likely (p < 0.001) than those at the other two clubs to have consumed any alcohol prior to the sweep interview, to anticipate more alcohol consumption, and to have engaged in any alcohol consumption at all over the course of the fieldwork night. Mean levels of consumption were also lower at the Leisure Centre than the other two clubs (p < 0.001). Customers in the Leisure Centre were least likely to report that on the fieldwork night they were mainly or only drinking (29.3 per cent compared to more than half in the other two clubs), and most likely to report that they were mainly or only taking drugs that evening (42.9 per cent compared to less than 20 per cent in the other two clubs).

Table 4.13   Alcohol consumption by club

Club	Warehouse		Leisure Centre		City Centre	
N = 2057	% any	(mean)	% any	(mean)	% any	(mean)
Mean alcohol:						
units consumed	87.7	(8.57)	57.1	(5.65)	89.0	(8.45)
units planned	71.5	(5.87)	52.1	(7.14)	67.1	(5.66)
Total	91.5	(12.19)	67.6	(9.73)	91.2	(12.08)
Consumption plans for evening:	%		%		%	
Mainly/only drinking	50.7		29.3		55.3	
Mainly/only drugs	20.6		42.9		16.8	
Both drinking & drugs	25.3		21.6		23.5	
Neither drinking nor drugs	2.5		6.2		4.3	

These differences in alcohol consumption by club are interesting for a number of reasons. The fact that respondents in the Leisure Centre were less likely to drink alcohol, and to do so in smaller quantities than respondents at the other two clubs, may in part relate to the younger average age of these clubbers. There was in fact a weak but significant relationship between age and alcohol consumption that occurred prior to the sweep interview, such that younger club goers were less likely to have consumed alcohol prior to entry into the club, and to have done so in smaller quantities than older respondents (although there was no relationship between age and planned consumption later in the night or over the course of the night). However, customers at the Leisure Centre, which of the three clubs was most similar to early 1990s 'rave'-style dance events, also voiced some of the negative attitudes held about drinking and drinkers in clubs discussed in Chapter 2, and thus their preference for a 'drug'- rather than 'alcohol'-orientated venue:

She voiced a concern that since the Leisure Centre has had a drinks licence, some people just go there to get drunk and cause trouble ... [and that] the Leisure Centre often gets a lot of drunks. She said that later in the evening she felt particularly unsafe in the car park where gangs of drunken lads cause trouble. (100403, 19-year-old female who drinks less than once a year)

And:

Pissheads were let in on 5th September ... big kickoff afterwards. Man in a wheelchair was hit with a bottle and was bleeding. (130203, 25-year-old male who drinks several times a year)

Even amongst some of the frequent drinkers, alcohol consumption at clubs was viewed as problematic:

He feels safe in clubs in terms of his drug taking, but worries about aggression from drunk people. He has suffered in clubs from the over-reaction of drunk men that he has accidentally knocked into. (021119, 21-year-old male who drinks daily)

And:

He doesn't like the drinkers who go to the Leisure Centre (or 'wankers' as he called them) because of the violence they cause. (130709, 16-year-old male who drinks daily)

Respondents at the Leisure Centre also mentioned some of the negative effects that alcohol had on them:

He complained of drink being more trouble, especially to him as he has a very bad allergic reaction. He becomes violent after drink and it makes him very ill, or alcohol poisoning reaction after only a couple of drinks. Even his mother prefers him to take drugs than alcohol due to the effect it has upon him. (110506, 30-year-old male who drinks several times a year)

I want something nice served at the bar – not alcohol or water, not something with vitamin C in it because it brings me down from my drugs. (130203, 25-year-old male who drinks several times a year)

These differences in alcohol consumption by club are connected to the cultural and ideological perspectives associated with the 'decade of dance' discussed in Chapter 2. Whilst age may be significant in that younger clubbers were somewhat less likely to have been drinking prior to coming out, and to have done so in smaller quantities than their older counterparts, both were equally likely to drink over the course of the evening and to anticipate similar levels of consumption. Essentially clubbers at the Leisure Centre exhibited some of the 'alcohol negative' sentiments of the late 1980s and early 1990s associated with the acid house and 'rave' culture, which emphasised the 'luv'd up' 'happy vibe' associated with ecstasy use in particular. Whilst anti-alcohol sentiment existed at the other two clubs, it did not appear to the same extent and was not, given the rates of purposeful drinking in these venues, necessarily related to actual consumption anyway.

Drug repertoires on clubbing nights

Continuing the analysis with the large club sweep survey sample, Table 4.14 details drugs which respondents had already taken and were planning to take on the fieldwork night. Alcohol consumption was on the agenda for more than eight in ten clubbers (64.8 per cent), and two-thirds would consume one or more illicit drugs.

Table 4.14   Drugs clubbers had already taken and were planning to take on fieldwork night for selected drugs in the club sample (N = 2057)

Drug	Had already	Had/planning to:
(Alcohol)	78.2	83.6
Cannabis	33.8	42.2
Ecstasy	26.1	36.1
Speed	28.4	31.8
Poppers	4.4	8.6
Cocaine powder	4.9	6.8
Legal herbal drugs	5.2	6.2
LSD	1.6	2.2
Tranquillisers	0.3	0.9
Viagra	0.4	0.8
GHB	0.6	0.6
Heroin	0.2	0.2
Crack	0.0	0.1
At least one (not including alcohol)	56.6	64.8
Number of drugs taken on the fieldwork night		
None		35.3
One		22.2
Two		22.3
Three		14.0
Four or more		16.3
Mean		1.36

In terms of individual drugs, we deal first with the ubiquitous cannabis (Forsyth, 1998). As we have seen from their drugs histories (Table 4.4), the majority of clubbers have ever taken cannabis (more than eight in ten), and have taken it recently (about seven in ten). Their cannabis use routinely takes place during the day or evening prior to going out (33.8 per cent), often as part of the ritual of preparing to go out (see Table 4.14). It also has a pivotal role as post-clubbing 'chill out' drug as we discuss shortly. These cross-contextual qualities ensure its high prevalence.

Moving to the key dance drugs, ecstasy (36.1 per cent) and amphetamine (31.8 per cent) continue to be the staple choices of clubbers as they have been across the last decade whether in Wales (Handy et al., 1998), Northern Ireland (McElrath and McEvoy, 1999), Scotland (Hammersley et al., 1999) or England (Release, 1997). Whilst the demonisation of ecstasy has had an impact on a cohort of mid-adolescents at the end of the 1990s (Aldridge et al., 1999; Balding, 1999), it has had little impact in clubland, as it remains the most popular drug of choice outside of cannabis.

We must be careful not to confuse the rapid growth in the recreational and 'partying' role of cocaine (Corkery, 2000; Boys et al., 1998) with its specific use in dance clubs and night clubs. Its use is clearly on the increase in clubland, with just under 7 per cent taking it on their clubbing night out. However, factors including price, method of ingestion and the relatively short lasting effects (resulting in 'topping up' requirements) may well prevent it becoming a dance floor favourite.

Poly drug use was common. Only just under one-quarter of the sample (22.2 per cent) either took or planned to take only one drug on the fieldwork night. The average number of drugs taken was 1.36. More than half of clubbers in the sweep sample (52.5 per cent) were taking two or more drugs on the fieldwork night: just under one-quarter (22.3 per cent) took two drugs, 14.0 per cent took three drugs and 16.3 per cent took four or more drugs.

We also see some interesting differences in drugs used by gender and age (see Table 4.15). Women were significantly less likely to be taking an illicit drug (57.5 per cent) than men (70.7 per cent) on the fieldwork night. And for each drug individually, where gender differences existed, use on the night out was more prevalent amongst men. These gender differences held for cannabis (34.2 per cent for women compared to 48.8 per cent for men); for ecstasy, taken by about one-quarter (26.9 per cent) of women compared to under half (43.7 per cent) of men; poppers, by about 1 in 20 women compared to about 1 in 10 men; and LSD, taken by 0.6 per cent of women compared to 3.5 per cent of men. Amphetamine was the only dance drug for which rates of use by males and females were equal.

Table 4.15   Drugs clubbers had taken/were planning to take on fieldwork night by gender and age (N = 2057)

Drug	M	F	sig	15–17	18–20	21–25	26–30	31–57	sig
(Alcohol)	83.3	84.0	ns	71.4	83.3	85.6	83.2	82.7	ns
Cannabis	48.8	34.2	***	46.9	41.9	45.9	35.2	41.8	*
Ecstasy	43.7	26.9	***	34.7	31.6	38.8	34.6	52.4	***
Amphetamines	31.9	31.6	ns	42.9	30.3	33.3	24.4	42.9	***
Poppers	10.7	5.9	***	2.0	5.9	8.8	14.3	11.8	***
Cocaine	8.8	4.4	***	4.1	3.7	8.8	8.4	11.8	***
Legal herbal drugs	7.0	5.2	ns	2.0	6.4	6.7	5.0	7.1	ns
LSD	3.5	0.6	***	4.1	2.5	1.7	1.9	3.5	ns
Tranquillisers	1.2	0.6	ns	0.0	0.2	0.9	2.2	2.4	**
GHB	0.9	0.2	*	0.0	0.4	0.2	0.3	4.1	***
Viagra	0.7	0.9	ns	0.0	0.9	1.1	0.0	1.0	ns
Heroin	0.2	0.3	ns	0.0	0.1	0.2	0.9	0.0	ns
Crack	0.1	0.2	ns	0.0	0.1	0.2	0.3	0.0	ns
At least one (not including alcohol)	70.7	57.5	***	67.3	60.6	70.0	58.3	77.6	***

Whilst ecstasy was more popular than amphetamines for men, the reverse was true for women. These findings again confirm significant differences in drug taking between women and men in clubs. Even though gender differences in overall prevalence rates have been narrowing amongst adolescents and in some club settings (e.g. Handy et al., 1998), the ways in which women and men use individual drugs continue to differ. We have already seen small but significant differences in lifetime and past three month prevalence rates, as well as in frequency of use rates, by gender. But these fairly small differences actually hide relatively substantial differences in day-to-day drug use. Although women in clubland tend on average to be younger than men, and to have initiated into drug use at a younger age than men, our findings suggest that fewer of them are taking illicit drugs in clubs than men (McElrath and McEvoy, 1999).

With respect to age, there appears to be no easily understandable pattern, although the majority of the sample (15–30) have some variations. There are some differences in drug choices and a tendency for the oldest clubbers to be taking the most drugs (particularly ecstasy and cocaine). There are few linear age-related patterns except for poppers and cocaine, in which numbers taking these drugs on the fieldwork night increases with age. One feature again to be emphasised is how the youngest clubbers appear very quickly to have developed dance drug repertoires which correspond with those of older and more experienced clubbers.

Table 4.16 illustrates these same statistics on drugs used on the night out but this time by venue. As indicated earlier, alcohol was least likely to be consumed at the Leisure Centre hardcore dance venue, by about two-thirds of club goers there, compared to over 9 in 10 at the other two clubs. However, use of at least one drug, simultaneously, was highest at this venue (76.6 per cent) compared to around 6 in 10 club goers at the other two venues. Use of cannabis was also highest at the Leisure Centre, as was use of ecstasy and amphetamines (this drug by about twice the number of club goers at the other two venues). Again, this highlights the early Nineties-style alcohol-negative, 'happy vibe' 'rave' ethos at this venue. This 'traditional' rave style is also illustrated in rates of cocaine use at the Leisure Centre, less than half (3.8 per cent) the rates of use of this drug at the other two clubs (about 8 per cent). This is also likely in part to be due to cocaine's status as an expensive and sophisticated drug, so it is unsurprising that its use was higher at the other two clubs, both city centre-based, and both with relatively high socio-economic, and older, customer bases. Use of poppers on the night was many times higher at the predominantly gay City Centre club (20.0 per cent) compared to only a small number of respondents at the Warehouse club (2.5 per cent) and the Leisure Centre (3.2 per cent). Again, these differences in drug use point to the variation in how drugs are used according to age, class and sexual orientation.

Table 4.16   Drugs clubbers had taken/were planning to take on fieldwork night for selected drugs in the club sample (N = 2057)

Drug	Warehouse	Leisure Centre	City Centre	Sig
(Alcohol)	91.5	67.6	91.2	***
Cannabis	44.0	53.9	28.9	***
Ecstasy	35.8	40.7	32.0	**
Amphetamines	23.1	48.0	24.9	***
Cocaine	8.2	3.8	8.3	**
Legal herbal drugs	6.2	7.4	5.0	ns
Poppers	2.5	3.2	20.0	***
LSD	1.6	3.0	2.2	ns
Tranquillisers	0.8	0.6	1.3	ns
GHB	0.4	0.0	1.3	–
Heroin	0.3	0.2	0.3	ns
Crack	0.0	0.0	0.4	–
Viagra	0.0	0.0	0.8	ns
At least one (not including alcohol)	60.5	76.6	57.6	***

Finally, the timing of consumption and the order were also affected by clubbers' intentions in the early hours. Although about half (52.2 per cent) of clubbers in the interview sample usually went home after the club, the remainder (47.8 per cent) intended to go on to other dance clubs, bars, breakfast clubs or house parties.

The ideal clubbing–drugs repertoires

We asked the dance drug sample to tell us what their favourite drug, or combination of drugs, was for a night out clubbing. Table 4.17 illustrates the drugs named by clubbers as their 'night out' favourites. For over three-quarters of the sample (78.0 per cent), ecstasy was named as one of their favourite clubbing drugs, and for over six in ten respondents, amphetamines were named. This points to the continuing stability and predominance of ecstasy and amphetamines in the clubbing repertoire over the last decade and into the next. And, consistent with the finding that only 6.8 per cent of respondents had taken cocaine on the fieldwork night, only about one in ten respondents (11.2 per cent) named cocaine as their favourite, or one amongst their favourite, clubbing drugs. Even where, presumably, cocaine is available and affordable, only a minority of club goers would nominate it as a favourite. Again, this suggests that new concerns about the use of cocaine in dance clubs may be somewhat misplaced. The fact that cannabis is named as a favourite clubbing drug by only 16.0 per cent of respondents further confirms its status as a generic drug; whilst it was the most commonly used drug on fieldwork nights its primary role remains off the dance floor.

Table 4.17   Drugs named by respondents as their favourite clubbing drug for the interview dance drugs sample (N = 317)

Drug:	%	Mean
Ecstasy	78.0	
Amphetamines	63.6	
Cocaine	11.2	
Cannabis	16.0	
All other drugs	8.9	
Number of drugs		1.7
One	38.5	
Two	53.7	
Three	7.4	
Four	0.3	

The majority of interviewees named two illicit drugs (mean 1.7) as part of their ideal repertoire, whilst just over a third (38.5 per cent) named only one. The remainder (7.7 per cent) nominated more than two substances. Remembering these drugs are, in most cases, taken in conjunction with alcohol, we are again describing a poly drugs repertoire (Handy et al., 1998).

The relative sophistication and specificity of dance drug use is further illustrated when we look at the typical chronological order of consumption (Table 4.18). Cannabis use before a night out is part and parcel of its general use, whereas its dominance as post-club 'chill out' drug is directly related to its relaxing properties and potential to induce sleep. This counteracts the stimulant effects of the dance drugs, including ecstasy which clubbers take just before and particularly inside the club, as well as amphetamines and cocaine.

Table 4.18   Typical order of consumption* for favourite clubbing drugs for the dance drug interview sample (N = 316)

	Before (%)	Inside (%)	After (%)	No specific order (%)
Ecstasy	44.0	63.4	8.6	17.7
Amphetamines	73.0	31.1	3.9	14.9
Cannabis	57.6	11.5	85.2	34.6
Cocaine	60.8	43.4	2.3	17.4

*Figures for 'before' and 'inside' each include respondents who typically took the drug 'both' before and inside the club.

Typical amounts of consumption for the sample were relatively moderate. On average, clubbers typically consumed 2.17 tablets of ecstasy over the course of a night out clubbing; 1.25 grammes of amphetamines; and 0.72 grammes of cocaine.[4]

Positive experiences of drug taking

The reasons ecstasy, supported by alcohol, amphetamines and cocaine, remains the clubbers' favourite drug connects with the hedonistic and spiritual motives of the first 'waves of rave' which sustained the 'decade of dance'. As Chapter 2 argues, integral to our understanding of dance drug use must be the physical, symbolic and cultural context for use. The setting: the club, the dance floor, the posing and posturing, the buzz of anticipation and excitement and, most of all, the music are all available to drinkers and abstainers; but with tablets and powders the fusion and enhancement of the experience and endurance therein are uniquely amplified. These dance drug users illustrate the significance of this:

Energy. Get in rhythm with the tunes. Bloody big smile on my face, confidence to approach people. I couldn't come out straight, it's not the same ... I love her loads but want to make the most of my life clubbing. If she asked me to choose between the drug and her I really don't know what I'd do. You only live once. (130203)

If the music is good it brings you up on the drugs – it's a two way thing. (060711)

I've been working hard all week – really hard and on Saturday nights it's my recreation and it's better than aerobics. (060705)

She felt it was difficult when you were into the music – because of media reports – if her parents heard her playing it they would assume she was on drugs ... She summed it up wonderfully with the phrase 'music is our football' – more important than drugs, but the two go together. (050804)

He questioned whether clubbing was a way of escaping. Rather, clubbing is life ... clubbing is our leisure time. It's better than booze. Everybody moves together. There's a consciousness. A consensus. A community ... Leisure the Nineties way of debauchery. (030319)

The respondent fits in well with others I've interviewed at the City Centre club so far – reasons for use being 'to be totally out of it' and 'dancing my tits off'. Tonight the reason given was 'Plan B – which is fuck it!' (180712)

We asked clubbers to tell us which amongst a series of positive effects they'd had during or after drug taking. Results (Table 4.19) suggest that clubbers identify a range of related benefits nearly all of which correspond with the effective use of their weekend 'time out' from everyday life and realities.

Table 4.19   Positive experiences during or after drug use for the interview sample (N = 362)*

Positive effects	N	%
Happiness	200	55.7
Energy	150	41.8
Dancing	129	35.9
Sociability	93	25.9
Time out/forget worries	90	25.1
Music	74	20.6
'Treat myself'	68	18.9
Confidence	65	18.1
Sexual excitement	54	15.0
Relaxation	40	11.1
Celebrate	39	10.9
Reduce stress	37	10.3
Habit	33	9.2

*3 respondents had missing data for this question

Discussion

There are certain groups of heavy alcohol users or problem drug users who have been extensively researched over many decades by both medical and social researchers. Writing about a new data set for such groups (e.g. alcohol dependants, problem heroin users) involves situating new findings in an established and well-known knowledge base. Issues of validity, representativeness and so on are relatively straightforward to address. This is not so for the clubbers and dance drug users for whom there is only a very small literature and thus limited knowledge base. Because they are poorly understood, our knowledge is thus particularly distorted by the media and intuitive constructions about clubs, drugs and 'trouble'.

We have already argued that the prospects for developing a good knowledge base are poor. It is unlikely there will be sufficient investigation of clubs and of those who frequent them to produce a reliable knowledge base. The difficulties – political, methodological and financial – in researching this arena are so substantive as to ensure this 'private' world of serious drinking and recreational drug use is likely to remain only partly understood. This makes writing about the results of this study difficult: to situate and pitch the conclusions or be able to demonstrate generalisability. So whilst the findings discussed in this chapter seem clear and robust and produce a convincing picture, there is always the worry that they cannot be compared with other investigations. For instance, we know of no other study which has specifically detailed the drugs careers of very young clubbers and focussed on their remarkably brief yet florid use of so many drugs as they eagerly enter the dance club–night club scene. The findings in this study are unequivocal about this particular drugs pathway but we have no scientific means of locating them in the 'literature' because it doesn't appear to exist.

The important point here is that it is to multiple structural, cultural and individual explanations that we must look, rather than simple mono-causal explanations. Clearly a social and cultural understanding of dance drug use (as discussed in Chapter 2) is important. In this study we have found that structural differences such as gender play a significant role in dance drug use. But at least in terms of who the clubbers are, there is a consensus amongst club research. Every study has found that they are young adults who come from a wide range of social backgrounds. We have found, similarly, that dance club customers in our three large venues were in the main between 18 and 30 years old, predominantly in their early twenties and from all socio-economic backgrounds. Whilst some clubs attracted a criminogenic element from the social margins, a key point is that those who were employed in higher education and from professional occupations were heavily represented. This is vitally important. If we are to understand and appreciate the attractions of drinking and taking Class A drugs and getting 'out of it' in fairly dramatic ways, we cannot call upon class-based or social exclusion-type analyses.

Whilst social and cultural factors must play a role, other clues can also be found in the clubbers' backgrounds: seven in ten were smokers, almost all were regular drinkers, and they had exceptionally high rates of early drug trying. Whether currently 'resting' from dance drug use or not, they were neither cautious nor conservative but were in academic terms 'sensation seekers' and 'risk takers', suggesting that for at least a proportion of these dance drug users it is with psychological and behavioural characteristics that we find commonality. The seasoned dance drug users will try new drugs like GHB or Viagra. They tread where more cautious peers will not.

A picture of young adults who should know better, embroiled in poly drug use, can easily be painted. The clubber as a smoking, drinking, cannabis-'dependant' and Class A drug user is an identikit picture easily constructed. And indeed, as we shall see in the next chapter, this is not wholly unreasonable as a significant minority pay a serious price for such psycho-active substance repertoires.

On the other hand, we see strategic decision making and hear articulate voices which suggest that the dance drug users, perhaps in part because they are economically productive, employed and/or educated citizens, are in control. They value their nights out in terms of socialising, dancing, exercising, cavorting, 'copping off', and taking intoxicated time out from the weekly grind. They generally steer clear of heroin and crack cocaine, most only take amphetamines and ecstasy at weekends and usually in moderate doses. They often self-medicate through their come-down period. They appear to employ rational cost-benefit decision-making strategies and include the role of alcohol in 'spoiling' nights out in these assessments. Their thresholds of tolerance are high and their assessments may seem risky to the majority of the (older) adult population but on the other hand they are far more self-disciplined than problem drug users of particularly addictive drugs (Power, 1995) and few get involved in drugs-acquisitive crime lifestyles.

This said, the potential for these serious recreational drugs careers to lead to problems with use and worse is there. In particular the identification of a very young segment of clubbers provides food for thought. The consequences of the normalisation of recreational drug use amongst 1990s adolescents are evident in this study. Some of those who became recreational drug users in mid-adolescence, across the second half of the last decade, have quickly moved into the club scene. We find 17- to 20-year-olds with extensive drug experience, gained at pace, almost immediately mimicking the dance drugs repertoires and clubbing lifestyles of older and more experienced clubbers which were built up over far longer time-spans.

In the next chapter we assess the costs of clubbing on physical and psychological health and the working week. It will be particularly important to see whether the youngest dance drug users experience disproportionate costs and/or lack the accumulated wisdom to minimise and mediate any unwanted consequences.

5 From Coping Strategies to Health Costs

The costs of commitment

In the last chapter we noted how committed to their leisure choice clubbers were. Whilst some young people simply pass through or occasionally 'visit' the clubbing phenomenon, most appear to be enthusiastic regulars. They go out frequently, they rate the experience highly, they spend a good deal of disposable income on their nights out and list a range of enjoyments and positives which they associate with dancing on drink and drugs.

Committed clubbing, because it involves strenuous physical exercise, endurance and public 'performance' bears some parallels with sport – for example professional football. In such sports, the best professionals often appear as precocious teenagers, have setbacks but generally reach peak form during their twenties, overcome injury and incident and survive into their thirties by compensating for reduced physical performance by acquired wisdom and 'reading' the game. Many others drop out of the sport through injury, loss of commitment and motivation, or an inability to cope with the lifestyle.

In this chapter we describe the various physical, psychological and health costs of a clubbing career as described by the dance drug-using interview sample (N = 317). Just as in sport, almost all clubbers require a recovery period from their weekend exertions. Most are able to cope with the negative physical and psychological experiences they perceive to be side-effects of their drug use, negatives which may be seen as analogous to the minor injuries, stresses and strains of the sport, but a minority experience more substantive problems with physical and psychological costs. A few report quite serious 'injuries', particularly in respect of incidents whilst on the field of play – the night out – and, it seems, more significant mental health problems with which dance drug use may be linked.

We describe the costs of clubbing through self-reported and medically assessed morbidity and produce what for some observers may appear a daunting list of negative outcomes. However, these negatives are mediated by the clubbers' social and psychological constructions of the costs of clubbing and their coping strategies employed to minimise negative outcomes. What for many may appear unacceptable risks and costs are to a large extent acknowledged and suffered by clubbers as the necessary price paid for the brilliance of nights out dancing on drugs.

Recovery from dance drug use

For the club goers in this study, the night out was a long and demanding one. The average length of stay in the club was almost four hours,[1] during which most clubbers will have spent a considerable proportion of their time in the exertions of dancing. However, as we have already seen in Chapter 4, for most club goers (about eight in ten), the evening began even earlier with alcohol consumption in bars, pubs or at home, and for about half of our clubbers, continued afterwards when they went on to other dance clubs, bars, breakfast clubs or house parties. With additional hours spent travelling to and from venues (see Chapter 6), we can see that the clubbing night out can easily last many hours longer than the four spent in the club. For most clubbers, therefore, we would expect that some sort of recovery period will be required, particularly and crucially because of the centrality of stimulant-based drug use to the clubbing night out.

Our dance drug users often spoke in their interviews of their 'come down' after their clubbing weekend (e.g., Curran and Travill, 1997), acknowledging the need for a recovery period and often striving to incorporate time for it within their working lives. One interviewer noted:

> He had very specific reasons for taking speed tonight ... he had not had anything for six months ... He had a week off work and felt he would have time to recover. (110316)

Another dance drug user, however, disputed the existence of a psychological/emotional come-down period: '[It's] mind over come down. If you're strong minded you don't have come downs.' However, he recognised the obvious physical consequences of taking drugs which acted to suppress the appetite. 'It takes a toll on your body. I was a bag of bones so I've cut down a bit.' (141103)

As can be seen in Table 5.1, very few of the respondents in the interview dance drug sample (2.6 per cent) stated that they typically required no recovery period whatsoever.

Recovery periods did vary considerably amongst dance drug users, but for most (about 80 per cent) it was confined to no more than a two-day period. The largest proportion, about one in three (35.6 per cent) took one full day to recover. For just over a quarter (26.5 per cent), the recovery period lasted longer, up to two days, and for about one in five clubbers (19.9 per cent), the recovery period lasted two days or more. The average length of the recovery period was 1.72 days, and the maximum number of days required for recovery was seven days, although for only 2.8 per cent of respondents. This suggests that for clubbers for whom the recovery period was one day or less (about half – 50.5 per cent), where the night out occurs on Friday or Saturday nights, recovery will take place during the course of the weekend when most are free from work or study commitments.

Table 5.1   Recovery period for the dance drug interview sample (N = 317)

	n	%	Days
None	8	2.6	
Less than one day	39	12.3	
One day	113	35.6	
> 1 to 2 days	84	26.5	
More than two days	63	19.9	
Mean			1.71
Median			1.00
Maximum			7.00

*10 respondents had missing or invalid responses to this question

However, for the remaining half, the recovery period may extend into the working/studying week, particularly when the night out occurs on a Saturday night. This will also be true for those clubbers who go out midweek and for those whose jobs involve weekend work, whereby the recovery period will be coinciding with those work commitments. Furthermore, those clubbers with responsibilities caring for children and dependants will not necessarily have the luxury of a weekend recovery period: there is a likelihood that any come down will coincide with carer commitments regardless of the day of the week they went clubbing. At a rough estimate, therefore, this suggests that *at least* half of our club goers will have recovery periods that overlap with work, study and carer commitments (see also McElrath and McEvoy, 1999). The comments of some dance drug users to fieldworkers confirmed this overlap:

It usually took him about four days to recover from taking drugs. He said this affected his work at university as he hardly ever goes in. (010405)

Another dance drug user, when talking about the recovery period, said 'I get up late and lose time sitting around doing nothing' (010206). One interviewer noted the effect of a dance drug user's weekend drug use on the working week:

It affects his work – 'always late, and looks and feels like shit' – but he said his bosses are all doing the same sorts of things so it doesn't put his job at risk. (071117)

In fact, our interviewees were asked directly if their weekend drug use or 'come down' affected their work or study in the week afterward. Table 5.2 shows that fewer than half (41.2 per cent) indicated that this was the case. If in fact our rough estimate is correct that about half of dance drug-using clubbers have recovery periods that overlap with work, study and caring responsibilities, it confirms our expectations that almost as many are actually reporting that their come downs affected their work, study or caring.

Table 5.2   The effect of the recovery period on work and study for the dance drug interview sample (N = 317)

	n	%
Affected work/study*	130	41.2
*Nature of effect:***		
Tired/fatigue	34	30.6
Performance/quality of work	34	30.6
Absent/time off/late	21	18.9
Mood swings/depression	20	18.0
Lack of concentration/memory loss	19	17.1
Hate day 'X'	15	13.5
Work relationships affected	6	5.4
Sacked/expelled	5	4.5
General health problems	4	3.6
Paranoia/anxiety	3	2.7
Improves work performance	6	5.4

*25 respondents had missing responses to this question.
** 9 respondents did not go on to specify the nature of the effect. Base percentage here is respondents who reported at least one effect on work or study (n = 111).

We asked all dance drug users who reported effects due to their come downs on their work or study to tell us the nature of the effect (see Table 5.2). The most common was fatigue and performance/quality of work (30.6 per cent) followed by absence from work, mood swings and lack of concentration (just under one in five clubbers). More than one in ten (13.5 per cent) clubbers reported that there was a particular day that they experienced the most difficulty with (most often the Monday, Tuesday, Wednesday after the weekend). One fieldworker noted during her interview with a dance drug user: 'Wednesday is usually a wash-out but by Thursday usually getting over weekend drug use' (0107805). Smaller numbers (5 per cent or fewer) reported that their relationships at work had been affected, that they had been sacked or expelled, general health problems, or paranoia and anxiety. Interestingly, about 5 per cent volunteered that their weekend drug use when clubbing actually improved their work performance.

Although these more serious effects – potentially and some actually damaging to health, work and social relationships – were rare, one interviewer noted a dance drug user who told of devastating effects on his work:

> He had also taken PCP [phencyclidine] on a weekly basis for a short time ... there was no order or predictability to his usage. 'Any – makes no difference. Just as it comes. Soon as I get it. Get the job fucking started.' His drug use 'totally destroyed' his work. 'Keep away from it 'cause they're bad' he explained with a huge slice of irony before adding 'but they're dead good!' (030319)

As we have seen, the length of the recovery period from dance drug use varied considerably amongst club goers. How can these variations be explained? The length of the recovery period could not be predicted by knowing dance drug users' demographic characteristics: it was unrelated to gender, age or sexual orientation. We might expect, however, recovery time to be related to the type, quantity or frequency of drug use. For the most part, though, this was not the case: the length of the recovery period was unrelated to the frequency of use or to typical quantities used for any of amphetamines, cannabis, ecstasy or cocaine. However, we did find that the length of the recovery period was related to the type of drug used and user status. Dance drug users who defined themselves as 'users' of amphetamine had significantly longer recovery periods (1.92 days) than dance drug users who did not consider themselves to be amphetamine users (1.54 days) ($p < 0.05$). Recovery time was also related to poly drug use. The greater the number of drugs respondents nominated themselves as users of, the longer the duration of the recovery period ($r = 0.173$, $p < 0.01$), although this relationship was not strong. This was also true for the number of only 'dance drugs' used (amphetamines, cannabis, LSD, ecstasy, poppers and cocaine) ($r = 0.149$, $p < 0.01$).

To a fairly small extent, therefore, we do find a relationship between drug-taking *behaviour* and recovery time from clubbing drug use, primarily in relation to whether respondents considered themselves amphetamine users, and in relation to having larger poly-drug use repertoires. This is an important finding in an area of little research into individual problems related to the growing trend in poly drug use.

We did find, however, that dance drug users who attached greater importance to clubbing had longer recovery periods (the correlation was small, $r = 0.157$, but statistically significant, $p < 0.01$). But although those dance drug users who attached a greater importance to their clubbing tended to go out clubbing more often ($r = 0.338$, $p < 0.001$), the length of the recovery period was not related to clubbing frequency ($r = 0.021$, ns). Thus, whilst self-reported recovery periods do vary considerably amongst dance drug users, those who went out clubbing more often were no more likely than those who went clubbing less often to report experiencing longer recovery periods.

Why do dance drug users for whom clubbing (and its associated drug use) is more important report experiencing longer recovery periods than those for whom clubbing is less important? It is possible that dance drug users who rate clubbing and its associated drug use as important to them focus more upon their experiences of that drug use, and pay closer attention to all aspects of that experience, including the 'come down' and recovery. Perhaps dance drug users define the physiological and psychological experience of the come-down period in different ways: those for whom clubbing and drug taking is important may attend to and therefore notice the nuances of their come down more than others. Thus, the dance drug user quoted above who stated, '[It's] mind over come down. If you're strong-minded you don't have come downs' (141103) is helpful in drawing our attention to the link between psychological 'set' and interpretation of the drug experience (see Zinberg, 1984), which may be extended to include interpretation of the experience of the come down. It may well be that there are also physiological factors and related differential rates of recovery for individuals which better explain their range of recovery time, but assessing these was beyond the scope of our study.

Negative experiences with drug use

We asked the sample of dance drug interviewees to nominate which of a wide-ranging list of physical and psychological negative effects or outcomes they had ever experienced during or after taking drugs (this list was adapted from Release, 1997). Their responses related primarily to cannabis and the dance drugs. As Table 5.3 demonstrates, most of the experiences we asked about were highly prevalent amongst our sample of dance drug users.

Fatigue (71.6 per cent) and insomnia (66.1 per cent) topped the list. Both of these we would expect to be common effects of stimulant-based drug use, in which fatigue results after a period in which users are unable to relax or sleep. Only a small number of dance drug users (1.9 per cent) had experienced no negative physical effects during or after drug taking. The average number of negative physical effects for the sample, out of a total of 11, was 5.04 (the median was 5). Although the least common in the sample, one in five dance drug users (20.1 per cent) had passed out or become unconscious during or after drug use.

Negative psychological experiences were also typical for this sample of dance drug users, although somewhat less so than negative physical experiences. All but 12.1 per cent had experienced at least one of the five psychological symptoms, and the mean number of symptoms experienced was 2.63 (the median was 3). Topping the list of negative psychological experiences was depression (62.0 per cent). Just over half of dance drug users had experienced amnesia (55.9 per cent), paranoia (55.0 per cent) and excessive mood swings

Table 5.3   Negative effects ever experienced during or after taking drugs for the dance drug interview sample (N = 317)*

Negative experiences	n	%
Physical experiences		
Fatigue/lack of energy	224	71.6
Insomnia	207	66.1
Blurred vision/dizziness	205	65.5
Weight/appetite problems	187	59.7
Nausea	174	55.6
Headaches	141	45.0
Stomach pain	134	42.8
Vomiting	127	40.6
Skin problems	86	27.5
Irregular periods (as % of females)	34	26.6
Passing out/unconsciousness	63	20.1
Psychological experiences		
Depression	194	62.0
Amnesia/vagueness	175	55.9
Paranoia	172	55.0
Excessive mood swings	169	54.0
Panic attacks/anxiety	115	36.7
Number of physical experiences:		
None	6	1.9
1–2	47	15.0
3–4	81	25.8
5–6	97	30.9
7–11	83	26.4
Number of psychological experiences:		
None	38	12.1
1	49	15.6
2	61	19.4
3	61	19.4
4	54	17.2
5	51	16.2
Mean number of 11 (max.) physical experiences		5.04
Mean number of 5 (max.) psychological experiences		2.63

* 3 respondents had missing data for this question

(54.0 per cent). Just over one-third (36.7 per cent) had experienced panic attacks or anxiety.

We undertook several interviews in which respondents disclosed dramatic psychological problems. Although comments such as these below were relatively rare, they do show that some dance drug users experience severe problems that they link directly to their use of dance drugs. This first interview was also discussed in Chapter 3 in relation to our professional responses:

> In a rush of openness he admitted that speed had led him to contemplate suicide and the depression (which he appeared to have sought no help for) lasted for at least six months … I could have caught him at a bad time, or on a bad night, but the overriding impression was of worry and vulnerability. (010803)

And:

> He worries about both his mental and physical health in the future and says there has been a permanent effect on his personality from his drug taking. He is now shyer and more introverted than he used to be, finding it more difficult to talk to people … He is convinced that in the future he will go 'downhill' because he will never stop taking drugs. 'I will end up in a psychiatric hospital, schizophrenic or something, definitely.' (020205)

Overall, these results suggest that the majority of dance drug users experience both physical and psychological problems associated with their drug use. What these analyses do not address, however, is the extent to which these negative effects associated with their drug use concern them. Do they perceive these effects as simply consequences of their drug use, to be both accommodated and accepted? Or do these negative effects associated with their drug use overshadow their enjoyment of their clubbing experience? We asked the sample what they disliked about taking drugs in clubs, using an open-ended question to which they could respond in any way. Answers to this question provide an insight into the relative priority of physical and psychological problems compared to other problems dance drug users associate with drug use in clubs. The results are contained in Table 5.4.

Table 5.4   'Dislikes' about taking drugs in clubs for the dance drug interview sample (N = 317)*

Concerns surrounding:	n	%
Policing & illegality issues	75	23.9
Psychological problems	64	20.4
'Nothing'	56	17.8
Social problems	21	6.7
Physical problems	14	4.5

* 3 respondents had missing data for this question

Individual reported problems were grouped into several categories: policing and illegality, psychological, social and physical.[2] Interestingly, although (as we saw in Table 5.3) almost all dance drug users (98.1 per cent) reported experiencing at least one negative physical effect associated with their drug use when prompted from a structured list, we see here that only 4.5 per cent of dance drug users spontaneously suggested that physical problems affected their enjoyment of taking drugs in clubs. This provides some evidence that the negative physical effects associated with dance drug use for most dance drug users do not overshadow their enjoyment of the clubbing night out. This is not to suggest that physical effects were not perceived as highly problematic for at least a minority of users and clearly some effects were quite serious. A fieldworker noted about one dance drug user, for example: 'Two years ago he had an allergic reaction to speed in which he bled from his ears and eyes' (010108).

A sizeable minority, about one in five dance drug users (20.4 per cent), identified psychological problems as affecting their enjoyment of drug taking in clubs. Although negative psychological effects appear to have a greater impact on the enjoyment of the clubbing night out than do negative physical experiences, given that nearly nine in ten (87.9%) experienced at least one negative psychological effect, this again suggests a sense of commitment to the dance drug experience in which enjoyment far outshines costs.

Finally, whilst we can conclude that quite real negative physical and psychological costs are endured by dance drug users that appear only to marginally affect their enjoyment of clubbing nights out, we must remember that our sample was made up of current dance drug users. When we look at our comparison interview sample we find a drug-experienced group of primarily ex-dance drug users. Between a third and a half had ever experienced the main physical symptoms of fatigue/lack of energy, insomnia, blurred vision/dizziness, weight/appetite problems, and nausea, and were just as likely as the current dance drug users to report having had negative psychological effects. In particular, they were highly likely (95.5 per cent) to report having cut down or stopped their use of one or more drugs. This all suggests that at least some club goers, having experienced too many 'negatives', decide to continue clubbing without dancing on drugs.

And finally, we should not forget that whilst morally comfortable with their drug use, nearly a quarter of dance drug users remained concerned about the law-enforcement agenda related to their drug use (23.9 per cent), the policing and regulation of their nights out and getting caught up in this in some way. These concerns are discussed at length in Chapter 6.

Coping strategies

Given the physical and psychological costs of being regular recreational dance drug users and club goers, combined with a commitment to the dance club scene, we should expect clubbers to apply coping strategies and techniques to avoid or minimise the various harms (Shewan et al., 2000; Akram and Galt, 1999; Branigan and Wellings, 1999; Branigan et al., 1997). We asked our sample of dance drug users how they avoided the problems they associate with their use of drugs. This question was open-ended so dance drug users could respond in any way. The results are found in Table 5.5.

Table 5.5   How respondents avoid the negative effects associated with their drug use for the dance drug interview sample (N = 317)*

	n	%
Do nothing	71	22.9
Drink well	74	23.9
Eat well	62	20.0
Change drug use – quantity consumed	40	12.9
Get sleep	39	12.6
Take other illicit drugs	35	11.3
Get support from others (friends, partner, family)	30	9.7
Take care over frame of mind	28	9.0
Relax/rest/'chill out'	28	9.0
Take vitamins	24	7.7
Take over-the-counter/prescribed medicines	15	4.8
Change drug use – timing/frequency	12	3.9
Take exercise	10	3.2
Change drug use – type of drug	8	2.6
Take care over environment	5	1.6
Drink more/less alcohol	5	1.6
Change drug use – quality control	3	1.0
Average number of strategies reported (mean)		1.3

* 7 respondents had missing data for this question

Over three-quarters of dance drug users (77.1 per cent) took one or more steps to avoid or minimise the negative effects they associated with their drug use. Ways that dance drug users generally 'took care' of themselves topped the list: eating well and drinking well (with more than one in five dance drug users nominating these tactics), along with getting sleep (12.6 per cent), relaxing and resting (9.0 per cent), and taking vitamins (7.7 per cent). These responses were typical: 'He takes vitamin C after taking acid, a good sleep after E and he is careful to eat properly' (010705); and 'He counteracted any adverse effects by a healthy diet and working out at a gym' (010405). Often users referred to getting support from others (9.7 per cent) and taking care over their frame of mind (9.0 per cent) (Shewan et al., 2000). Comments from a female dance drug user illustrate:

She has experienced negative effects from taking drugs including amnesia, panic attacks, depression and mood swings. To avoid getting any of these negative effects she said that she hides away from the rest of the world. She puts on the answer machine and stays indoors – 'disconnects from the real world'. (010708)

One of our fieldworkers, having interviewed in turn each of a male–female couple, noticed:

... a marked difference in their approaches in dealing with the possible negative effects of drug taking. He was interested in being proactive and preventative whereas she either dealt with it afterwards with some other drug (ibuprofen/antibiotics/alcohol) or didn't do much about it. (020505)

This quote reflects two styles of secondary prevention and coping tactics detailed in Table 5.5. One involves taking care of general health, well being and psychological or emotional state and the other involves drugs, for instance by modifying drug intake, changing drug of choice, quantities or styles of use, and also utilising over-the-counter pharmaceutical drugs. More than one in ten dance drug users (12.9 per cent) suggested that they changed in some way the quantity of their drug use, usually reducing their dosage to reduce the negative effects. One in ten (11.3 per cent) took other illicit drugs to alleviate symptoms, and 4.8 per cent did so with the use of over-the-counter remedies such as ibuprofen, aspirin or paracetamol. Smaller numbers mentioned other ways of changing their drug use, including the timing or frequency, changing the types of drugs taken, or changing their alcohol consumption in some way.

Thus most dance drug users adopt one or more from a range of tactics to avoid the negative experiences they associate with their drug use. They seek to minimise the negatives and maximise the positives, and often spoke of trading advice amongst friends that allowed them to take care of their own health and that of others. This comment illustrates:

She realises the health implications [of her drug use], perhaps more than most as a friend has died on methadone (non-prescribed) and a family member on solvents. Very matter of fact, she added later that she had saved somebody's life by giving the kiss of life at [another club] in [another town]. (010802)

We can also see that dance drug users are concerned about the potential effects of their drug use on their health and well being in the future. Over three-quarters of the dance drug interview sample (79.5 per cent) indicated that they had such concerns. Although not all went on to specify what their concerns might be, about one-quarter (23.4 per cent) indicated concerns for their physical health and a similar proportion (24.6 per cent) to their psychological well being. One-third (33.3 per cent) suggested that uncertainty about the effects on their future health and well being affected them. These varying concerns are unsurprising given the public health debate centring around MDMA that features frequently in the media and particularly in the music press (e.g., *Mixmag*, 1998), as well as scientific debate about neurotoxicity and MDMA that has continued since the beginning of the decade (e.g., Peroutka, 1990).

All this suggests that dance drug users do experience problems with their drug use, that most take steps to avoid problems, but that they remain concerned about their future health in relation to their drug use. Given that they appear to be proactive rather than passive in the management of their physical and psychological well being, this provides us with some evidence that dance drug users are a clear and receptive target for health education and harm reduction information. This harm reduction policy implication will be discussed in more detail in the final chapter.

A further gauge of problems with use is whether clubbers have cut down or stopped the use of one or more drugs. The majority of our interview dance drug sample (N = 317) reported having cut down or stopped the use of a drug (84.9 per cent). As we shall see, dance drug users moderated or stopped their drug use for a number of reasons. However, for a majority, this occurred because they experienced some aspect of their drug use as problematic, at least enough for them to take some measure to do something about it. As noted above, even more (95.5 per cent) interviewees in the comparison sample had cut down or stopped the use of a drug.

The drug most cited by those who had cut down or stopped was amphetamines (44.6 per cent) followed by ecstasy (30.0 per cent). Less frequently, dance drug users reduced or stopped their use of cannabis (16.5 per cent), LSD (15.3 per cent), and cocaine (7.3 per cent) (all as percentages only of those ever having tried each drug). Thus, consistent with much of what dance drug users told us in their interviews, the drugs they experienced the most problems with were amphetamines and ecstasy. This is unsurprising, given too that we found negative experiences during and after drug use were most often linked to use of these drugs, which were in any case the most used dance drugs.

Our interviews with dance drug users suggested a link between age, or more specifically, maturity and changing life circumstances, and cutting down or abstaining from certain drugs or drug repertoires. We found many examples of older and more experienced clubbers describing this process:

Generally I just don't need to take as much as I used to. I used to go out and have four pills and be out of my brain. Now I don't do more than 1½ pills. I can go home, go to bed and get up the next day because of the kids, one aged four and one aged 18 months. I don't need to get that out of it. That's your honeymoon period: taking as much as you can to go as far as you can. I've done all that and don't need to do it. (150206)

And:

She felt she had to stop whizz because 'her head would have fallen off'. (130810)

This theme of changing or cutting down on specific drugs as part of the maturation process is echoed in several interviews:

She has cut down on drugs before, stopping totally when pregnant, and she realises the health implications. (010802)

And:

He had to cut down on both ecstasy and speed and he attributed this to a raised awareness of potential dangers but also due to work reasons: he had a responsible job with good prospects and his days of 'driving round the city scoring' were over. (031114)

And another:

At 28 he considered himself a seasoned raver of the old school ... he has cut back a lot on drug taking although he can't imagine clubbing without anything. (100901)

However, quantitative analyses did not confirm this link. Most dance drug users in this study, regardless of age, had cut down or stopped taking at least one drug at some time in their drug careers. It is possible, however, that whilst age is unrelated to frequency and amount of drug consumption (as we showed in Chapter 4), older club goers may, when they were younger, have been heavier dance drug users than the current group of young clubbers. It could be, therefore, that in the early days of the ecstasy and dance club scene, as anecdotal evidence suggests, clubbers who are now in their late twenties and early thirties were consuming much more in terms of quantity and frequency than younger clubbers do now, particularly of ecstasy and amphetamines. The finding that most clubbers, regardless of age, appear now to be consuming similar (moderate) amounts may mask greater reductions in use that have occurred primarily amongst older dance drug users over their drug-taking careers.

Sometimes reasons for cutting down or stopping were linked to ideas about quality or purity, particularly in relation to ecstasy: '... too many bad pills going about' (100403), and sometimes harkening back to an earlier period when ecstasy was thought to have been better: '... they don't make them like they used to' (101101) and 'He started taking ecstasy seven years ago but does not take it now because it is not "real MDMA"' (010401). As we have seen in Chapter 2, this may reflect a nostalgia for days gone by when ecstasy in particular was seen to be purer and better. This nostalgia, both for the quality of the drugs and the quality of the dance scene, has been evident since shortly after the beginning of the 'decade of dance'. However, as we saw in Chapter 3, our urine analysis suggests that the ecstasy in particular taken by our dance drug users in the north-west of England was pure MDMA, surprisingly strong and unadulterated (although as we discuss in Chapter 3, some of our dance drug users appear to have been sold ketamine as ecstasy).

In summary, most dance drug users adopt a range of tactics and techniques to minimise the negative outcomes associated with their drug use. They appear to balance out the negatives with the positives, and with experience and by sharing information learn to cope with the downside of serious recreational drug use (Shewan et al., 2000).

Factors associated with negative experiences from drug use

Demographic predictors of negative experiences with drug use

What characteristics of individuals predict the negative effects dance drug users report having with their drug use? We turn our attention now to gender, sexual orientation and age. Table 5.6 summarises (only the) statistically significant relationships of these outcomes to various demographic measures.[3] As we shall see, gender and age in particular were associated with negative experiences with drug use.

All significant analyses by age showed that dance drug users who had each negative experience had a younger mean age than those who did not (t-test) and that age was negatively correlated with numbers of negative experiences (Pearson's 'r').

Gender was a significant predictor of negative physical effects during or after taking drugs. Female dance drug users were significantly more likely to report having suffered from nausea (63.3 per cent compared to 50.3 per cent of males) and headaches (52.3 per cent compared to 40.0 per cent for males), and also on average reported significantly greater numbers of negative physical effects during or after taking drugs than male dance drug users (a mean of 5.4 symptoms compared to 4.8 symptoms for males). Whether female dance drug users actually experience more negative effects related to their drug use, or whether they are simply more aware of these effects, and/or more likely to report them, we cannot tell. There were no gender differences, however, in negative psychological experiences.

Table 5.6   Statistically significant relationships between negative effects ever experienced during or after taking drugs, and gender, sexual orientation and age for the dance drug interview sample (N = 317)

Negative experiences	Male	Female	'Straight'	Gay/ lesbian	Bisexual	Age
Physical experiences						
Fatigue/lack of energy	–	–	–	–	–	–
Insomnia	–	–	–	–	–	–
Blurred vision/dizziness	–	–	–	–	–	–
Weight/appetite problems	–	–	–	–	–	**
Nausea	*50.3	*63.3	–	–	–	–
Headaches	*40.0	*52.3	–	–	–	–
Stomach pain	–	–	–	–	–	**
Vomiting	–	–	–	–	–	–
Skin problems	–	–	–	–	–	–
Irregular periods	–	–	–	–	–	*
Passing out/unconsciousness	–	–	–	–	–	–
Psychological experiences						
Depression	–	–	*57.9	*75.9	*70.0	–
Amnesia/vagueness	–	–	–	–	–	–
Paranoia	–	–	–	–	–	**
Excessive mood swings	–	–	–	–	–	–
Panic attacks/anxiety	–	–	–	–	–	–
Mean no. of 11 (max.) physical experiences	*4.8	*5.4	–	–	–	***
Mean no. of 5 (max.) psychological experiences	–	–	–	–	–	*

3 respondents had missing data for this question
p < 0.05; ** p < 0.01; *** p < 0.001

Those dance drug users who described their sexual orientation as gay/lesbian were substantially more likely to report having suffered from depression during or after taking drugs than heterosexual dance drug users (75.9 per cent compared to 57.9 per cent).[4] Again, we cannot determine the extent to which gay and lesbian dance drug users may simply be more aware of, or willing to report, their depressive states, or whether they actually experience more depression. This finding linking depression with sexual orientation may alternatively suggest that it is possible that drug use may exacerbate pre-existing depressive states. For one gay male dance drug user, drug use represented a form of 'self-medication' or psycho-active time out that may in part have been related to stressful experiences that included public acknowledgement of his sexual orientation:

> [His] father was on a life support machine ... he hasn't seen him for six or seven years ... he had testicular cancer ... he was a prosecution witness in a murder trial ... At this time he was 'coming out' [as a gay man] so it was a very traumatic time. He was on six anti-depressants ... and he goes clubbing and takes drugs to forget about everything. (190721)

The most significant demographic predictor of negative effects experienced during or after drug use was age, with younger users experiencing more problems than older users. Table 5.6 shows that dance drug users who experienced weight/appetite problems, stomach pain, irregular periods and paranoia, were all more likely to be younger than dance drug users who did not experience these effects. There were also significant negative correlations between numbers of negative physical experiences ($r = -0.192$) and psychological experiences ($r = -0.115$) and age, such that younger dance drug users reported significantly more of both kinds of symptoms than older users. These findings confirm that older dance drug users experience fewer problems in relation to their drug use. The most likely explanation for this finding is that older dance drug users may have learned more effective ways of avoiding negative effects, and the data in fact support this hypothesis. There was a significant positive correlation between age and number of strategies employed (see Table 5.5) ($r = 0.12$, $p < 0.05$), such that older dance drug users tended to employ more strategies than younger ones to deal with the negative effects of dance drug use. This suggests that older dance drug users may have more information available to them regarding how to deal with the negative effects of drug use, have a wider bank of experience upon which to draw, and/or are more willing or able to implement strategies. All this strongly suggests the importance of the cumulative effects of years of drugs 'education', via dance club culture, drugs agencies and the media, combined with becoming 'drug wise' and learning through their own and friends' experiences (Parker et al., 1998). Again, this finding has relevance to secondary prevention messages.

Behavioural predictors of negative experiences with drug use

Table 5.7 contains the significant relationships between negative physical and psychological experiences and whether respondents considered themselves to be users of selected drugs.

Dance drug users who considered themselves to be ecstasy users reported suffering from the most negative consequences during or after drug use, both physical and psychological. Ecstasy users reported significantly more negative physical experiences (a mean of 5.6 compared to 4.4 for non-users of ecstasy),

Table 5.7 Statistically significant relationships between negative physical and psychological experiences and whether respondents considered themselves to be users of selected drugs for the dance drug interview sample (N = 317)

	Amphetamines Non-user	User	Cannabis Non-User	User	Ecstasy Non-user	User
Physical experiences						
Fatigue/lack of energy	–	–	–	–	**61.8	**78.7
Insomnia	**59.0	**76.5	–	–	–	–
Blurred vision/dizziness					***54.2	***73.8
Weight/appetite problems	**52.2	**71.2	*51.7	*65.4	–	–
Nausea	–	–	–	–	–	–
Headaches	–	–	–	–	**35.1	**51.8
Stomach pain	–	–	–	–	–	–
Vomiting	–	–	–	–	*33.6	*46.3
Skin problems	–	–	–	–	–	–
Irregular periods	–	–	–	–	–	–
Passing out/unconsciousness	*16.3	*25.8	*14.2	*24.0	–	–
Psychological experiences						
Depression	–	–	–	–	*54.2	*68.3
Amnesia/vagueness	–	–	**45.8	**64.2	***41.2	***68.9
Paranoia	–	–	–	–	–	–
Excessive mood swings	–	–	–	–	*47.3	*60.4
Panic attacks/anxiety	–	–	–	–	*29.0	*41.5
Mean no. of 11 physical experiences	**4.7	**5.4	**4.6	**5.4	***4.4	***5.6
Mean no. of 5 psychological experiences	–	–	*2.4	*2.8	***2.2	**3.0

Base percentage is dance drug users who had ever tried each drug. Only 14 dance drug users considered themselves to be users of LSD, so numbers were too small for analyses. Numbers were also small for cocaine (37). No significant relationships were found for cocaine, although this will at least in part have been due to the relatively small numbers of users. LSD and cocaine are both excluded from presentation in the table.

and reported suffering disproportionately from fatigue, blurred vision, headaches and vomiting. Ecstasy users also reported significantly more negative psychological experiences (a mean of 3.0 compared to 2.2 for non-users of ecstasy), and reported suffered disproportionately from depression, amnesia/vagueness, mood swings and panic attacks/anxiety.

In contrast, amphetamine users were not significantly more likely than non-users to report negative psychological experiences during or after drug use. This may in part be due to the fact that amphetamine sulphate is a physical stimulant, whereas ecstasy is considered to be an empathogen or stimulant hallucinogen. However, amphetamine users had more negative physical experiences (a mean of 5.4) than non-users of amphetamines (mean of 4.8), and were more likely to have experienced insomnia, weight/appetite problems and unconsciousness.

Being a cannabis user was also predictive of problems experienced with drug use (see McGee et al., 2000). Cannabis users reported significantly more negative physical (mean of 5.4 compared to 4.6) and psychological (mean of 2.8 compared to 2.4) outcomes related to their drug use, and specific negative experiences included both physical symptoms (weight/appetite problems) and a psychological one (amnesia/vagueness). Problems with forgetting and vagueness were typical amongst cannabis users. One interviewer noted:

> The respondent regularly used cannabis until he quit completely because it had become a problem. He said he had 'lost nine months' of his life through heavy use. Cannabis had affected his memory and he was constantly tired. (010401)

We also examined the relationships between negative experiences with drug use and frequency of drug use (see also Hammersley et al., 1999). Frequency of use was related to negative experiences for only one drug, cannabis, and this was for only one negative experience – blurred vision/dizziness. Cannabis users who reported experiencing blurred vision/dizziness had an average reported frequency of cannabis use of 5.5 times per week compared to 4.4 times per week for cannabis users not reporting this problem. Frequency of use of ecstasy and amphetamines was unrelated to individual physical and psychological problems. Furthermore, there was no relationship for frequency of use of any of the three drugs and numbers of physical or psychological problems reported, although clearly the dance drugs tended not to be used as frequently as cannabis in these clubbers' repertoires (see Chapter 4). However, the fact that frequency of use for ecstasy and amphetamines was unrelated to physical and psychological effects may be an artefact of how we measured these effects. Dance drug users were asked if they had *ever* had any of the negative effects we listed. We were unable to address, therefore, the extent to which these experiences were current, ongoing, or particularly problematic. It appears that negative effects represent very common symptoms of dance drug use, even if moderate or infrequent. These symptoms, therefore, may simply be part and parcel of dance drug use.

We explored the relationship between reported problems with drug use and quantities of drugs used. The quantity information was gathered by asking dance drug users for their favourite combination of drugs taken on a night out, along with ideal amounts. Although this may not reflect actual amounts used on a typical night out, it does represent a useful gauge of quantities consumed. Amounts were coded as numbers of grammes ideally consumed over the course of the night for amphetamines, cocaine and cannabis, and as numbers of tablets for ecstasy. Only 25 dance drug users in the interview sample listed cocaine as one of their ideal drugs for a night out and provided ideal quantity information for the drug. Results for this drug are therefore not discussed.

Negative effects with drug use were most often related to quantity of ecstasy consumed, although some relationships were found for quantity of amphetamines and cannabis. Two negative physical effects linked by dance drug users to their drug use were related to quantity of consumption of ecstasy. Having been unconscious or 'passing out' was associated with greater quantities of ecstasy ideally taken on a night out (an average of 2.7 tablets compared to 2.1) as was having vomited (2.4 tablets on average compared to 2.0). Two negative psychological effects were also found to be related to quantity of ecstasy ideally consumed. Dance drug users reporting excessive mood swings had higher average consumption (2.4 tablets compared to 1.9 tablets), as did users reporting amnesia/vagueness (2.3 tablets compared to 1.8 tablets). There was also a small but significant positive correlation ($r = 1.6$, $p < 0.05$) between numbers of negative psychological effects reported and ideal amounts of ecstasy consumed, such that those with higher consumption tended to have more negative psychological effects.

Dance drug users who had experienced weight/appetite problems ideally chose to consume 1.4 grammes of amphetamines compared to 1.0 grammes for those who had not. Also, dance drug users who had experienced amnesia/vagueness reported higher amounts of cannabis consumption on a night out (3.5 grammes) than users who did not (1.2 grammes).

Dance drug users with larger poly drug use repertoires reported experiencing more negative physical ($r = 0.267$, $p < 0.001$) and psychological ($r = 0.233$, $p < 0.001$) symptoms.

Numbers of negative physical and psychological effects reported by dance drug users were unrelated to frequency of clubbing, and unrelated to whether or not dance drug users considered themselves to be regular clubbers. However, the younger dance drug users were when they began clubbing regularly, the more negative physical effects they experienced.

Symptoms experienced by dance drug users were also related to age of initiation of use of certain drugs: the younger dance drug users were when they first took the drugs, the more likely they were to have had more negative physical and psychological effects. There were significant negative correlations between negative effects and age of initiation into use of amphetamines, ecstasy, poppers and cocaine (all correlations were small, ranging from -0.125 to -0.188, but statistically significant at $p < 0.05$ or better). This is consistent with the finding discussed above in which younger dance drug users reported more negative effects with their drug use; not only do older drug users experience fewer negative effects, therefore, it also appears that the older dance drug users are when they begin taking dance drugs, the less likely they are to experience these effects.

The complexities of co-morbidity

Co-morbidity or 'dual diagnosis' is a highly complex phenomenon. Given the high rates of mental illness and psychological distress in the general population and in 16- to 19-year-olds in particular, along with the presence of alcohol and drug problems in this specific population (Meltzer et al., 1995), it is hardly surprising that we have identified a significant number of clubbers with both high levels of alcohol and drug intake and psychological problems.

There are numerous different mechanisms and pathways to co-morbidity (e.g., substance use may exacerbate pre-existing psychiatric disorder (Crome, 1999)), and we have probably identified several of them from the in-depth interviews. However, as the fieldwork notes below illustrate, untangling the aetiology and the significance of regular dance drug use remains difficult:

> His sickness is some sort of mental health problem – he believes he is possessed by an evil spirit that talks to him and he also believes he has been abducted by aliens. His doctors see his mental health problem (schizophrenia?) as in part caused by excessive dependent amphetamine use *but only in part*. The respondent is very proud that the doctors and psychiatrist have conceded another element too. His friends however see it all as simply amphetamine psychosis and they think he's improving because he's cut down. (110201)

We cannot, in the end therefore, move beyond describing the presence of co-morbidity which has not been identified in most other studies of clubbers although, in truth, most have not attempted to measure mental health anyway. Clearly an underlying mental health problem or psychological morbidity is likely to predict more negative experiences with dance drug use just as heavy stimulant or hallucinogenic drug use may trigger psychological distress. What we cannot really explore is the prevalence of the different mechanisms and life journeys to co-morbidity, or the aetiology involved.

Problems leading to medical interventions

So far we have discussed self-help and self-medication strategies utilised by clubbers to mediate the negative experiences associated with certain drug use. As we have seen, these negative experiences were common across the board and to a certain extent, therefore, may be inevitable 'symptoms' of dance drug use which must be accommodated and accepted, although mediated through self-help. We turn our attention now to the problems associated with drug use that have led to medical interventions, in an attempt to further gauge the extent to which dance drug users may be coming to actual or perceived harm resulting from their drug use. We include alcohol in this assessment both because the vast majority of our interviewees go pubbing as well as clubbing and because they routinely mix alcohol with their dance drugs.

Over their going out careers, 20.7 per cent of dance drug interviewees have been seen at a hospital Accident and Emergency Department for an injury sustained at a pub or club (see Table 5.8). Most injuries were as a consequence of fights and assaults (39.7 per cent) and alcohol intoxication-related injuries (29.4 per cent) such as falls, consistent with other research (Marsh and Fox Kibby, 1992; Shepherd, 1990). Men were more likely to experience these outcomes (25.3 per cent) than women (16.4 per cent).

Table 5.8   Problems with alcohol/drug use leading to medical interventions for the dance drug interview sample (N = 317)*

	n	%
Seen at hospital A/E department for pub/club injury	74	20.7
For problems linked by respondents to drugs/alcohol		
Seen by doctor	82	22.9
Seen at hospital A/E department	39	10.9
Seen by paramedics/first-aid staff at club	38	10.6

* 4 respondents had missing data for these questions

Nearly half (48.3 per cent) of our dance drug users reported that they experienced health problems that they linked to drugs or alcohol. However, not all sought medical intervention: 22.9 per cent consulted with their doctor, 10.9 per cent had been to hospital, and 10.6 per cent received attention from paramedics/first-aid staff at a club. Some dance drug users described health problems that they linked to their drug use for which they sought medical help:

> He has gone to the doctor when suffering from depression, anxiety and panic attacks. He didn't tell the doctor about the drugs but made the mistake of saying he's always felt like this. She wanted to refer him to a psychologist but he didn't fill in the forms and cut down on his drugs instead. (200104)

And:

> She used to take loads of drugs, but had a nervous breakdown and doesn't any more ... She stopped using cocaine and ecstasy and speed because she 'lost control of her life'. She was diagnosed with severe clinical depression and was in and out of hospital. She became bulimic and went down to six stone. (010105)

There was no relationship between either gender or sexual orientation and these outcomes. However, those who had been seen by paramedics at a club were substantially younger (21.2 years) than those who had not (24.2 years) (p < 0.01). As most of these were found amongst the younger clubbers at the Leisure Centre (13.2 per cent), the only club with first-aid staff on hand, this finding may in part be artefact: in our sample, it was the younger clubbers who had this facility available to them. However, it is likely that this finding may be more to do with inexperience with drugs than age. For those who had been seen by paramedics at a club, their first time usage of amphetamines, LSD and ecstasy were significantly more recent than those who had not been attended to by paramedics at a club. This suggests that novice users, rather than younger users *per se*, were more likely to come into contact with paramedics at clubs. The drug most cited as having been taken in these instances was ecstasy (52.0 per cent) followed by amphetamines (20.0 per cent). The top two reasons for presenting to medical staff at clubs were becoming unconscious (27.3%) and having breathing problems (15.2 per cent).

We will return to this casualty rate in the final chapter when we explore how it might be reduced and managed more effectively.

Viagra

One significant achievement of the project concerned a 'surprise' finding that Viagra was being used without prescription in the club scene, only a few weeks after the licensing of the drug for use in the UK in September 1998. A short report published by the *British Medical Journal* (Aldridge and Measham, 1999) in paper and electronic form prompted a national debate amongst health care professionals, academics, and the general public.

During fieldwork in the City Centre club, interviews conducted with staff and customers revealed that illicit supplies of Viagra were readily available in the club for £10 (50mg tablet). We immediately amended our interview schedule to include asking questions about the use of Viagra for the larger club sample as well as more detailed questions for everyone who said that they had used it. Based on 519 revised brief sweep interviews, responses confirmed that Viagra had been used as a recreational drug (i.e., not prescribed to them) by 15 respondents (2.9 per cent) (10 males, 5 females; 14 white, 1 African-Caribbean; mean age 26, range 19–34).

Of concern was the combination use of Viagra and other recreational drugs. Most reported having taken Viagra simultaneously with illegal drugs (MDMA, cocaine, cannabis), illicit drugs (amyl nitrite, GHB), and with alcohol. Amyl nitrite was of particular concern as it is contraindicated for use with Viagra, potentially leading to a dangerous drop in blood pressure. Although this is stated clearly in the product information leaflet, recreational users of Viagra are highly unlikely to have access to this information or to the advice of their GPs.

We decided to go 'public' early, before publication of any other findings from the study, given our public health concerns in relation to the combination use of Viagra and amyl nitrite in clubs. A report was published (Aldridge and Measham, 1999), and at the instigation of the editors on their rapid response website (eBMJ) was accompanied by a press release.

The health of the medical sub sample

Body Mass Index

Analysis of the medical sub sample suggests that a considerable proportion of our dance drug users are underweight, and under the norms for the UK population (see Table 5.9).

Table 5.9   A comparison of (%) distributions of Body Mass Index (BMI) between UK adults and the medical sub sample (N = 53)

Body Mass Index (BMI)	< 20 underweight	20.0 – 24.9 normal	25.0 – 29.9 overweight	>/= 30 obese
UK adults aged 20–65 years				
Males (1, 2)	7	50	36	6
Females (1)	12	54	25	9
Medical sub sample (N = 53)				
Males	26	61	13	0
Females	36	50	14	0

Sources: (1) Knight (1984) and (2) Jones et al. (1986)

As we can see, none of the dance drug users in the sample were in the obese category, although 6 per cent of males and 9 per cent of females in the UK population are obese. Substantially fewer of the dance drug users were overweight (13 per cent of males compared to 36 per cent in the UK; 14 per cent of females compared to 25 per cent in the UK population). More than half of our dance drug users (61 per cent for males and 50 per cent for females) were in the 'normal' weight category, slightly more than are of a normal healthy weight in the British population.

However, roughly one-third of females (36 per cent) and one-quarter of males (26 per cent) were underweight, considerably higher than the proportions in the UK population (12 per cent of females and 7 per cent of males). This finding is of concern, although it does not surprise us given the regular use of stimulant drugs in the sample (which in the hours and days after use can suppress appetite), and the exertions of sustained periods of dancing for these regular clubbers. However, whilst a considerable proportion of male and female dance drug users may be suffering potential ill-health effects due to being underweight, this must be balanced against the finding that more of our dance drug users are not suffering ill-health effects from being overweight.

Winstock (2000) has highlighted concerns about seriously underweight clubbers and purposeful dieting via stimulant drug use. Consistent with this, we found that about six in ten (59.7 per cent) of the dance drug interview sample said that they had experienced weight or appetite problems in relation to their drug use (see Table 5.3 above). Although only a small number of dance drug users indicated that one of their reasons for taking drugs on the fieldwork night was to lose weight (1.3 per cent), it is likely that a much higher proportion have done so in the past or do so on other occasions, or certainly identify and 'enjoy' their slimness as a consequence of stimulant use and clubbing.

Analysis of blood and urine in the medical sub sample

In-depth medical assessments were carried out by an independent medical centre at the University of Manchester. From the dance drug interview sample 53 respondents have complete data from these assessments (see Chapter 3 for a discussion of the representativeness of this sub sample). In all cases where abnormalities were observed by medical staff, GPs were notified with respondents' consent.

The results of these tests are detailed below.[5] In summary, however, we found that about one-third of the sub sample had blood tests suggestive of anaemia, and more than one in ten had blood tests suggestive of infection. Worryingly, about one in five of the sub sample had urine tests indicating starvation, suggesting they had not eaten for at least a day or two.

Haematology
About one-third (17–32.1 per cent) of the medical sub sample had haemoglobin levels below the normal range, and of these, 15 (28.3 per cent) had additional abnormalities that indicate pointers to anaemia. Only three, however, (5.7 per cent) had clinically significant anaemia, with haemoglobin levels of < 12g.

Of the sub sample seven members (13.2 per cent) had mild leucocytosis (increased white cells) accompanied by an increase in the neutrophil subset of cells, indicative of a current infection.

Urinary Ketones
A striking 11 cases (20.8 per cent) had urinary ketones reported, and for none of these cases could this be explained as being due to diabetes (i.e., none had elevated blood glucose levels or glucose in urine). This is likely to be explained by starvation resulting from not eating for at least a day or two. This is a worrying result, and consistent with our finding that a considerable proportion of respondents were underweight.

Liver function/alcohol misuse tests
Abnormalities possibly due to excessive drinking were identified in two cases (2–3.8 per cent), although there were no other profiles suggestive of alcohol misuse.

Mildly raised bilirubin was found in seven cases (7–13.2 per cent), although none of them had any other liver function abnormality. It is possible that these raised levels are due to a mild toxic hepatitis. It has been suggested that ecstasy use may cause hepatitis.

Blood in urine

Six cases (6–11.3 per cent) were positive for blood in urine, and two were highly positive. Four of these were female and may have been menstruating.

Discussion

Most clubbers need a period to recover from their long nights out. Indeed, even if one didn't drink alcohol and imbibe drugs, the impact of a long night and physical exertions on the dance floor would usually be felt the next day. Over half of our dance drug sample, most of whom were also drinking, saw the next day as a natural recovery period beyond which they had few uncomfortable or unwanted after-effects. However, we have found that for nearly half our sample the recovery period is significant and overlaps with work or study. We have not fully understood why a significant minority are more likely to report fatigue, midweek depression, reduced performance, and so on, although we know that gender and age in particular play a role. Part of the answer may also lie in physical attributes and also, we suspect, in psychological perceptions of post-clubbing symptoms. Differences in reported recovery times are not easily related to patterns of drugs consumption, although there are indications that those in our sample who defined themselves particularly as ecstasy users, and those with larger poly drug repertoires, reported experiencing significantly more symptoms.

Whilst some of these symptoms are predictable and relatively benign, there are signs of significant morbidity, especially in respect of psychological disfunction. This said, and despite suffering a daunting list of negative outcomes, the majority of our dance drug-using interviewees did not see these as spoiling their enjoyment of clubbing. They tolerated and accepted outcomes such as fatigue, weight loss, midweek lows and so on as part and parcel of dancing on drugs.

Clubbers do employ harm reduction techniques and coping strategies and our sample was no exception. Most had one or more strategies ranging from having healthy diets, taking vitamins and getting exercise and rest, to more specifically reviewing and cutting back their alcohol and drug intake, and recognising the link between psychological state and a successful night out and the importance of social support.

Whilst women, gay men and lesbians appear to be more likely to report experiencing one negative psychological effect (depression), we have, in particular, found that being a younger and relatively novice drug user correlates with higher rates of negative outcomes. Incidents requiring medical attention were also more often disclosed by younger clubbers. Younger clubbers were also more likely to have no purposeful coping strategies, and at best, fewer than older clubbers. A further characteristic of younger clubbers is that the earlier their age of initiation with the key drugs, the more likely they were to suffer negative physical and psychological difficulties. These are important findings given our analysis (in Chapter 1) of how quickly adolescent recreational drug users move into the club scene as a consequence of the normalisation of recreational drug use during the 1990s and routine access to clubland from the age of about 17.

A major difficulty in this field of study is mapping aetiology. Because today's clubbers pick 'n' mix between the licit and illicit, and are increasingly likely to be poly drug users, we cannot satisfactorily isolate the effects of alcohol as opposed to cannabis, or amphetamines as opposed to ecstasy. We have shown how some of our analyses can highlight how *those describing themselves* as amphetamine or ecstasy users and who take high doses report more negative outcomes, but these analyses are insufficiently sophisticated to fully explore the impact of the consumption of such a range of psycho-active substances in varying combinations and over a wide range of time-spans. With the literature on clubbers pointing to poly drug use as the norm, it seems unlikely that either social or medical research, despite growing efforts, will be able to fully tease out the causal factors related to the long-term effects of dancing on alcohol and drugs in the foreseeable future.

A further example of the limitations of using clubbers as a study group has emerged in respect of examining co-morbidity. We have undoubtedly identified mental health problems in the dance drug-using sample, but cannot satisfactorily explore the aetiology from our fieldwork data. Our self-report data on negative effects have to be considered within the framework of interviewees using these drugs on the fieldwork night, and issues of self-perception and self-presentation in the semi-public interview setting of a club. But given the scale of mental health problems in the 16–25 age group, it was inevitable in such a large sample of clubbers that we would find psychological distress and symptoms of mental illness. What we cannot say beyond that there will be several different types of linkage and chronology is exactly what these are. We have probably identified morbidity independent of clubbing effects, triggered by drug use and even being 'medicated' by drug use but we cannot satisfactorily demonstrate this.

In policy and practice terms the shortcomings in our aetiological sophistication are not disabling. As we discuss in the final chapter, a secondary prevention–harm reduction agenda for clubland can be upgraded on the basis of our findings. For instance, it is enough to know that a minority of clubbers do suffer from a significant range of negative outcomes including psychological distress in order to review and upgrade secondary prevention programmes. First, however, we must explore 'health' in a rather different way, via the health and safety paradigm. In the next chapter we thus focus on how safe and secure clubland is, how dangerous going to town and getting home on weekend nights can be, and how clubbers obtain their illegal drugs and negotiate enforcement and the policing of clubs and drugs. As we have seen, many dance drug users do not like the fact that their drugs of choice are illegal. We can now explore how they deal with this contingency given their commitment to dancing on drugs.

6 Play Spaces – Safe Places? Violence, Safety and Security in Clubland

Having considered socio-cultural, consumption and health perspectives on dance drugs and dance clubs in previous chapters, we now turn our attention to issues of regulation, safety and security. In this chapter we will consider young people's acquisition of illicit drugs, aspects of supply and illegality, and related issues of drug distributors or 'dealers', violence and intimidation. The various perspectives and strategies surrounding drug distribution held by clubbers, club management and the police will be considered. Reported experiences of violence and intimidation in dance clubs and on the streets outside them raise issues of perceptions of safety and security which will be explored, alongside the policing and management of clubland. Finally methods of transport to and from clubs are discussed in relation to safety both on the streets and on the roads, for both clubbers and other transport users.

The elusive 'dealer': dance drug distribution and the law

As we saw in Chapter 2, some of the popular and media images of dance club culture have included the portrayal of dance clubs as dens of vice with drug 'dealers' ready to prey on 'innocent' young male and female victims (Henderson, 1993c; Redhead, 1993), echoing the association of night clubs and dance venues with drugs, sexual availability and general immorality going back to Britain's first dance drug underground in the 1920s (Kohn, 1997). Such images of club drug 'dealers' portray local 'gangsters', together with club staff, as central to a dance drug distribution network and wider dance scene which is characterised by violence and intimidation of clubbers (Swanton, 1998). We shall consider the extent to which this was true in our three north-west dance clubs as we explore the realities of recreational drugs distribution and issues relating to the policing of this widespread criminality.

Firstly, we assess the financial scale of drugs purchased to support a night out clubbing. Our interview sample of young clubbers (N = 362) reported having spent on average a total of about £51 on their whole night out the last time they went out clubbing (median £45), which included admission, soft and alcoholic drinks, food, cigarettes, transport and drugs. Looking at spending on drugs in particular, our interview sample estimated they spent an average of

£130 on drugs in the month prior to interview (median £70). The dance drug interview sample (n = 317) estimated that they spent about £18 specifically on illicit drugs on the fieldwork night (median £13), that is to say that about a third of the cost of a club night was spent on illegal drugs. In dance clubs with a capacity of about 800 customers such as the Warehouse and the City Centre clubs we might estimate from our findings in Chapter 4 that about half (400 customers) would take illegal drugs. If 400 people spent about £18 on drugs, it is apparent from even this rough calculation that one night in one dance club alone could result in over £7,000 worth of expenditure on illegal drugs. The temptations of large tax-free profits for distributors are also apparent.

Secondly, we look at how clubbers obtain their drugs and from whom. Of the dance drug users in our interview sample (N = 317) eight in ten (79 per cent) had paid for the drugs they were having on the fieldwork night and another two in ten (22 per cent) had received their drugs for free. Only 6 per cent of the dance drug sample received their drugs that night on credit and 1 per cent said they were traded or exchanged in some way. (Figures add up to more than 100 per cent because some poly drug users obtained different drugs consumed on the fieldwork night from different sources.)

Researchers have shown that despite the perceptions of the media, popular commentators, the public and (some) police officers of drug 'dealers' as part of 'Mr Big' mafia-style monopoly drug cartels, British drugs supply comprises a variety of different types of drug distribution enterprises. Law-enforcement policies tend towards smaller, decentralised and relatively 'disorganised' enterprises being more likely to stay in operation for a longer period of time than large-scale, centralised, highly organised monopoly drug distribution enterprises (Ruggiero, 1994; Dorn and South, 1990). 'Smaller is safer as far as drug distribution enterprises are concerned' (Dorn and South, 1990, p. 176). If we consider Dorn and South's classification of drug distribution enterprises and in particular three of the drug distribution types they identify – retail specialists, mutual societies and trading charities – we can use these three distribution types as a basis to explore our findings on dance drug distribution, similarities and differences to these three 'ideal' types, and wider issues of management, policing, violence and intimidation.

Retail specialists

Retail specialists are organised drug distributors working primarily for profit. Respondents discussed in considerable detail their general experiences of drug retail specialists at dance clubs. A typical operation was of known 'dealers', that is known both to the customers and the staff of a club, operating an agreed distribution within that club with several employees or 'runners' working for the manager(s) based in one corner. These runners specialised in their different tasks such as smuggling drugs into the club, acting as salesmen or 'snarlers', carrying the drugs and the money, distributing individual purchases to customers and collecting money, and acting as lookouts and minders. Such an operation might be condoned or sanctioned to a greater or lesser extent by staff working in that club. We identified retail specialists in all three clubs with door staff at one club, bar staff at another club and customers at a third observed by the research team involved in the purchase and provision of illicit drugs. This was further confirmed in conversations and interviews with customers.

One of the enduring images of clubland drugs distribution is that these retail specialists or organised drug dealership 'gangs' in clubs are more likely to sell poor quality or even fake drugs than if clubbers buy their drugs elsewhere before the event (Newcombe, 1992b; Saunders, 1993). Clearly there are unscrupulous people who take advantage of the anonymity of clubs and the enormous potential for profit mentioned above, in order to 'rip off' clubbers who want to purchase drugs (or more drugs) once inside a club. We interviewed one such self-confessed 'rip off' merchant in the course of our study. He told the interviewer:

> He had been arrested the previous week in Milton Keynes [leisure centre used regularly for largescale hardcore 'rave'-style dance events]. He said that he had been selling paracetamol – pretending that they were E's – to 'muppets'. He was charged with possession with intent and was awaiting further information. (090605)

Where regular clubbers at dance venues became familiar with a sanctioned or condoned club 'dealer' the situation was perceived differently from unknown 'dealers' in unknown clubs. On the whole, many customers approved of this regular small-scale individual club dealership because their regular presence and the informal sanction of club staff meant there was a degree of accountability. The chance of receiving poor quality or imitation drugs was minimised, as was the possibility of getting 'ripped off' by unscrupulous 'dealers'. As clubbers and 'dealers' pointed out to us, drug distributors who wanted to operate a profitable regular drugs outlet had a vested interest in satisfied customers who would return and purchase their drugs from them again the following weekend. Security staff at the club might sanction a particular operation or even guarantee an exclusive franchise in return for a certain percentage or 'taxing', thus providing added security for both the drug distributors and customers, whilst also minimising retail competition (Newcombe, 1992b; Fraser et al., 1992). Although clubbers acknowledged that they often paid slightly higher prices to purchase drugs inside the club, it was still possible to purchase good quality drugs, as has been suggested from the analyses of urine collected from our three north-west clubs discussed in Chapter 5.

The higher costs of in situ drug deals were explained to us in relation to the greater risks, level of organisation, numbers of individual employees and 'taxes' paid out to run a club drug dealership compared with a home-based dealership. Clubbers perceived a further advantage of the in-club deal rather than the pre-club deal in that the drugs were not carried by the individual clubber beforehand, therefore minimising the risks of being caught in possession on the streets, in pre-club feeder bars or upon entry into the club. The problem of carrying illegal drugs on the person and the risks of possession were mentioned by several respondents. If not buying drugs inside clubs, concerns about the risks of possession resulted in clubbers adopting strategies to avoid detection which even included burying drugs! One interviewer noted how:

> Intriguingly the respondent hides his drugs in a plastic bag 'outside the car' around the area. It appeared to be that he hid it around where he lived under a tree or something ... they are careful to not carry their drugs on them for any longer than necessary. (110313)

We interviewed several retail specialists including one ecstasy dealer who completed our full research programme: the dance drug interview, medical observations in the club, urine sample and the full medical at the university medical centre at a later date. He discussed how he prefered to sell ecstasy from home but because he was a known 'dealer', both clubbers and door staff still approached him and asked to buy drugs from him when he went to clubs:

> He said that since the [...] club had shut he had mainly been dealing at home. He did sell in clubs but this was because a lot of people knew him and approached him. He bought his pills for about £3 each and sold them for £10. I wondered about the safety of selling in clubs and he revealed he was from a local 'gangster' family and so knew most of the bouncers. Indeed they would often buy a load of drugs from him especially in [one of our three clubs]. With clubs closing in the city he felt the gangsters were cutting their own throats. He reckoned they were now moving on to new patches in a different city and were finding this relatively easy. (150801)

Indeed for some clubbers, the problem was not one of aggressive club 'dealers' being too pushy but being too elusive. One male respondent said to the interviewer during the sweep survey when he first entered the club that he hoped to consume dance drugs on the fieldwork night if he could obtain them inside the club. The interviewer wrote:

> When I did the initial sweep he hadn't had anything but was hoping/planning to get something somewhere somehow! He had been successful which led to

a long chat later on about how he knew who was selling and how reliable and safe the drugs would be. He said you get a good feel for who are dealers by their body language and position in the club but he agreed that approaching and asking strangers can be a bit risky. (030906)

Further purposeful observations by our research team throughout the course of the fieldwork confirmed organised drug distribution in each fieldwork club. One observation of suspected drug sales is given as an example here:

I saw what looked to me like a lad selling Es in the toilets. As I walked in a lad of about 20 was picking pills out of one hand with the other whilst another lad looked at these choices. Neither seemed to be too bothered by my or anyone else's presence. (090601)

It should be noted, however, that drug distribution was not overt in any of the three clubs. On the contrary, by and large it was the customers rather than the retailers who appeared to be more overtly proactive in making contact. Clubbers' searches for drugs retail specialists can be illustrated in the experiences of all research team members being approached on numerous occasions throughout the fieldwork period by clubbers asking to purchase drugs or asking for help in locating drugs retailers within the club.

The regulation of retail specialists

Strategies by club managers to deal with these drugs retail specialists in their clubs varied. The manager at the Warehouse club was willing to work with the police to control organised criminals who might intimidate clubbers and staff, although he was sceptical about the possibility of eliminating all drug distribution from his club. Just prior to our fieldwork, plain-clothes police officers visited city centre clubs with sniffer dogs with the aim of identifying the areas within clubs where drug sales might be occurring, in order for management to introduce more surveillance of the drug-dealing corners. One of the research co-ordinators attended the police dog search of the Warehouse club. The Warehouse club already had CCTV cameras inside the club at various points around the bar, dance floor and dark corners which had been identified as possible locations of 'trouble' of various sorts. There were also signs on the walls throughout the club saying that drug use would not be tolerated and anyone caught in possession of illegal drugs would be detained and the police called. The reality was that the police were not called to every incident of drug use discovered by Warehouse staff. One night one of the co-ordinators observed staff telling male clubbers to put away their cannabis and related paraphernalia. This was considered unusual by the clubbers and led to speculation about the door staff's action:

I was sitting down in the chill out area by myself at about 12. All the seats were taken but because it wasn't that full there wasn't anyone standing up. I saw two door staff go up and tell some blokes not to roll a joint and put it away. The door staff said they shouldn't be so open about it when it wasn't that full in the club and anyone walking in could see them skinning up. The blokes said to me that they usually don't have any problem rolling joints in the club, but it's usually much fuller and you can't see individual people as clearly as on this night. So overt drug use was being discouraged more than usual. (Co-ordinator fieldwork notes)

An hour later the door staff's keenness to discourage open cannabis smoking was put in context by police attendance at the club. It was not clear to the researchers whether this particular police presence was routine, a special operation or a raid and the club staff also did not appear to know whether it was routine or a raid:

At about 1am the police came into the club. I heard clubbers saying that the door staff said licensing people planned to visit the club that night and that might be a reason the door staff were clamping down on open drug use. Were these the licensing police, drugs squad or others? Did the door staff know the operation was going to take place? About ten uniformed police men and women entered the club and swept through the club in a quiet, low-key way and left with what seemed like a considerable number of people (from my restricted viewpoint). There didn't seem to be much conversation, opposition, resistance, signs of struggle or use of force. I didn't see anyone physically manhandled or handcuffed. Clubbers appeared to leave with the police of their own accord. It didn't seem to be a systematic raid, the police didn't talk to anyone near my patch of the club or systematically sweep through the club. The police didn't appear to have time to talk to people or assess who they were going to take away. It almost seemed like the police knew who they wanted and the men who left with them knew as well, they only had to be politely asked once to accompany them. The music didn't stop and the lights didn't go up. People stopped dancing for a bit and watched, then carried on dancing when the police left. A few people walked around looking a bit worried afterwards but most people just got on with the night. (Co-ordinator fieldwork notes)

Most weekend nights the police swept through the Warehouse club, doing a lap of the club and leaving. These police operations took the form of about seven to ten uniformed police officers from Tactical Aid based at a nearby police station making a brief appearance at 12 or 1am, sweeping through the club, walking round the perimeter of the dance floor, sometimes stopping to watch the dance floor for a few minutes, having a brief word with the duty manager and leaving. These Tactical Aid officers wore padded bullet-proof vests and were invariably white men in their thirties and forties. With the exception of the incident above, they did not usually apprehend anyone from the club on the nights that we observed them.

One night one of the co-ordinators talked to the police officer in charge of this Tactical Aid squad. The officer explained that the squad went to several city clubs in a night's work, turning up unannounced. After jokingly saying, 'We're like the Spanish Inquisition, we just turn up and make our presence felt', he went on to confirm there were two main aims. Firstly, it was hoped that the police presence would reassure 'genuine' clubbers and secondly, they wanted to stop, search and arrest known gun-carrying 'gangsters' who, it was believed, intimidated club staff and customers and extorted free drinks and admission. He said Tactical Aid knew who they were looking for, they knew their faces, it was quite specific people they were looking for; management at the Warehouse club confirmed this extortion, saying that aside from firstly, standard paying customers, secondly, the guest list and thirdly, the guaranteed entry list, there was also a small number of 'gangsters' who walked in without paying. 'You always get a few of them, especially at jungle nights, you just expect it and write it off', said the duty manager (see also Swanton, 1998.)

The co-ordinator asked Warehouse staff what their feelings were about these regular police midnight marches through their club. The duty manager said she was:

Happy for the police to routinely come into the club and for there to be a police presence in the club because 'it puts the wrong people off. It reassures genuine clubbers and puts off the gangsters.' (Co-ordinator fieldwork notes)

Other strategies at the Warehouse for the regulation of retail specialists and related problems included varying closing times. For example the monthly jungle night closed at 2am rather than the usual 3am on week-nights because it appeared to reduce the likelihood of trouble. The thinking behind this was that the local 'gangsters' did not see it as a big night out, just a minor weekday club night, so reducing the likelihood of trouble 'kicking off'. It is interesting to note that the jungle night was not particularly profitable for the club but club management said they were willing to take the risk of trouble, despite the lack of profits, as a marketing strategy. For many months the Warehouse club was the only dance club in the city to hold a jungle night. Management saw it as a symbol of their dominance of clubland, a statement of their confidence in their security operations and a stake in being one of the 'key players' in the city's nightlife. The duty manager explained:

The Warehouse wants to be seen to be at the forefront of this city's dance clubs and run a night like that but I'd prefer it if it was something else than jungle because it does always attract a certain element. I will have extra staff on the door that night and men also walking around inside the club to keep an eye on things and stop people smoking [cannabis]. But what can you do if they refuse to stop smoking, especially if lots of them are doing it? There's only a handful of door staff so they're outnumbered. And I have to think about their safety and not asking them to put themselves at unreasonable risk. (Co-ordinator fieldwork notes)

Alongside early finish times and extra security staff, the duty manager discussed one of the ultimate strategies in the struggle against trouble: prematurely closing the club on a problematic night, seen as effective in terms of policing if not business. The duty manager discussed a small group of 'gangsters' who were seen to get increasingly out of hand in the city, leading to the 1998 club clamp-down by police which was in operation during the fieldwork period. The duty manager discussed the circumstances of closing the club on one particular house music night when a group of local men

stormed the doors of various clubs around town including the Warehouse. Danny Rampling [national dance DJ] was playing that night and it was the first time he'd played this city for a long time because of previous trouble and we'd just persuaded him to do his first return gig. There were about 15 of them who went to the Warehouse that night and were being generally intimidating, and there wasn't much the six or so door staff could do. The police couldn't do much because they weren't really breaking any major laws, so I ended up just putting the lights on and shutting the club early. There's no way I'll let a bunch of black inner-city 17-year-olds spoil everyone else's night out. (Co-ordinator fieldwork notes)

The manager of the City Centre club was involved in the Pub and Club Watch scheme which represented all of the several hundred pubs, clubs and bars in that city. He was particularly outspoken about the issue of drug distribution and organised crime in clubland and critical of the police for their lack of involvement in policing the city centre clubs. He claimed that the number of pubs, clubs and bars in the city had trebled in the late 1990s but there had been no corresponding increase in police staffing to cope with the repercussions of this. He took a strong personal stance against organised crime and refused to allow the local 'gangsters' to intimidate him:

Born and brought up in the inner city ... he said he's seen some of the gangsters around the city since they were kids and he's not scared of them.

He said their aim is to scare people, not to fight them and that if you stand up to them they don't carry out their threats. He said he'd been threatened with guns, knives, fists, everything, on lots of occasions and has just challenged them and they've always backed down. If they were going to do anything, they'd have done it by now. He said the ones to watch are the ones that don't threaten you first. By contrast he felt that some club managers were their own worst enemies as they took the threats seriously and let themselves be scared, that their fear of gangsters was much worse than the reality of the threat. (Co-ordinator's fieldwork notes)

The City Centre club manager explained that he would like to see drugs decriminalised and sold in dance clubs like the one he managed, partly for financial motives but also for quality assurance and to disempower the organised criminals operating the retail specialist drugs chains in the city:

He described himself as 'anti-drugs': not that he particularly minds people taking drugs to enjoy themselves but he minds where all the money goes to, i.e. the criminal drugs gangs. He would like to see drugs decriminalised but wouldn't want people to buy their drugs outside the club and then the club not make any money from drinks. So he would like clubs to have a 'Pharmacy' counter located inside the club where they could buy quality assured drugs and the club could get the profits. He said he would be naïve to claim that there's no drug use in the club but he can claim with good reason [confirmed from other sources] that there are no dealers in the club. He's proud of the fact that the club has a reputation for no dealers. (Co-ordinator fieldwork notes)

On the issue of free admission and free drinks he took a stronger stance than the Warehouse club and was not prepared to 'write off' such extortion:

He had had gangsters coming in to the City Centre club and asking for free drinks, free admission, etc., and he always refused. He said to them they couldn't have free drinks and if they beat him up they still wouldn't get free drinks. He said his friend, the manager of another city centre club, once gave some gangsters a couple of free bottles of champagne and thought it would keep them sweet and get them off his back – by the end of the night they'd had 18 bottles. So he won't give them an inch on point of principle. (Co-ordinator's fieldwork notes)

We should bear in mind, however, that these three dance venues are not representative of all British dance clubs, nor even all north-west clubs. There are local and regional variations affected by policing, targeting and enforcement, as well as changing patterns of drug distribution and drug use which must be placed against the backdrop of broader socio-cultural changes in the British dance scene. Our fieldwork occured in 1998 and should be set in the historical context of the late 1990s/millenial debate surrounding 'gangsters' in clubland (see for example Reynolds, 1998; Garratt, 1998; Swanton, 1998; Haslam, 1999). Indeed, the three fieldwork clubs in many ways might be considered atypical because the managers agreed to allow us into their clubs and demonstrated their willingness for their clubs to be open to academic, public and police scrutiny. The manager of the Warehouse club said that he was willing to work alongside the police, drugs agencies and us too, if it helped to make the club a better, safer place. He reflected the pragmatic realism of many dance club managers in his concern to run a club free from violence and intimidation rather than attempting what he saw as the impossible: trying to run a club free from drug distribution and drug use.

Nevertheless, club management did express some concern about the implications of involvement in our research for their relationship with the police. The circumstances of the closure of a city centre club the previous year had been a turning-point in police/club relations, leading to strained inter-agency relationships and strong feelings on all sides. This added to the sensitivity of the timing and focus of this research project:

The City Centre club manager said his main concern in relation to our research was the police. He was very suspicious of the police, and did not trust them. When I said that the police had assured us that they would not target clubs that participated in the research or use the information to raid or close them, he kept saying the police don't always keep their word. He gave the instance of last September [1997] when the licences were revoked for the [...] club and the [...] club. He said that last September was the low point where morale hit rock bottom for club staff in the city and since then no one has trusted the police. Apparently the [...] club tried to work with the police, videoed inside the club for years and handed over all their videos to the police. The police said they would help the club sort out trouble and intimidation in the club but then used the five years of videos as evidence against the club at the hearing to revoke their licence last year. Other club management saw this as a big set-back to police/club relations too. 'If you co-operate with the police you get closed down, if the police say they'll help you they close you down.' (Co-ordinator's fieldwork notes)

Concerns about becoming the focus of police attention through club participation in our research were also expressed by other club managers. When the plain-clothes police inspector and two other police officers turned up to our very first fieldwork night the club manager described it as a 'planned coincidence'. This was despite assurances to us from senior police officers in the city that the police would not attend clubs on fieldwork nights. It was not clear whether the police presence on the first night indicated there had been a breakdown of communication between different police divisions, or whether they thought perhaps we needed protecting ... or policing!

In general the management at the three clubs were keen to discourage retail specialists establishing themselves in their clubs and to this end worked with the police for more efficient control of organised crime. Of particular concern was a small group of local men who attempted to gain free entry and free drinks through intimidation. Although these men were considered to be retail specialists, it was their attempts at extortion rather than their drug sales which were considered problematic. For this reason club management facilitated both uniformed and plain-clothes police operations within clubs on a regular basis. Management's willingness to operate alongside the police to ensure a safer atmosphere in clubland was tempered, however, by an awareness that the police presence would only be tolerated to a certain extent by clubbers on a night out. What club management did not want was harassment of their (drug using) customers, either from the 'gangsters' or from the police. They also did not want their requests for police assistance in their club to be used as ammunition for later closure of the club. Retail specialists did operate in the clubs, however, and in some cases with the knowledge and assistance of door and bar staff. This was evident in the numbers of respondents we conducted sweep surveys with as they entered the club who said they planned to have drugs on the fieldwork night if they were able to 'score' in the club. They were then interviewed or observed later in the evening, evidently under the influence of drugs and also confirming to us that they had been successful in procuring drugs in the club.

Mutual societies

A second form of drugs distribution is the mutual society or friendship network of user–dealers, defined by Dorn and South as users who sell or exchange drugs with each other in a reciprocal fashion. These drugs co-operatives or networks were evident in our study by the numbers of clubbers who admitted both giving and receiving drugs via friends. We asked our interview sample both whether they had ever received illegal drugs from friends, either free or for money, and whether they had ever given or sold illegal drugs to friends. It is interesting to note that 91 per cent of our interview sample reported having received illegal drugs from friends, either free or for money and 78 per cent of our interview sample reported having given or sold illegal drugs to friends. This finding has added significance in relation to current debates surrounding the Misuse of Drugs Act and the suggestion to introduce a new type of supply charge to acknowledge these mutual societies (Independent Inquiry, 2000).

There are considerable advantages to these friendship networks of user–dealers. Firstly, there are the obvious financial economies of scale of buying in bulk and missing out the middle level of drug distribution. Secondly, there is a greater security in making group drugs purchases, resulting in fewer individuals in contact with higher level drug distributors and less chance of theft of cash or buying low grade/fake drugs. And for those who were younger, less confident or less familiar with the world of drugs distribution, mutual societies might enable the less active members of the network to purchase drugs through friends without coming into direct contact with retail specialists themselves, although the more active members of the friendship network obviously would be making such contact. Thirdly, contact with other users facilitates sharing experiences and upgrading street wisdom regarding the effects of specific drugs and specific batches of drugs. Fourthly, friendship networks save time by reducing individual searches for supplies, a key issue in the hunt for the elusive 'dealer', particularly for those young adults with limited access to transport. Respondents discussed being able to take their time over the course of the preceeding week to obtain good-quality supplies from a reliable source – preferable to anonymous and unaccountable 'dealers' in clubs if the respondents did not regularly attend specific clubs with regular dealerships. Leisurely purchase in the preceding days or weeks might also facilitate the tasting or testing of drugs before purchase, if a considerable amount was being bought and they were regular customers. Fifthly, clubbers who discussed these friendship networks focussed on more than just the financial and time-saving aspects of group deals. A key feature was also the sociability and camaraderie of group drug purchases and consumption.

Thus friendship networks of user–dealers could also be considered to enhance three different aspects of harm minimisation. Firstly, by collective purchases made ahead of the night out, clubbers were able to make considered purchases of potentially better-quality drugs, resulting in less chance of adverse side-effects, after effects or long-term effects resulting from variable/fake street drugs, therefore minimising those health risks specifically associated with poor-quality drugs. (As we have seen in Chapter 5, however, adverse effects can also result from consuming the intended drugs.) Secondly, their contact with regular known 'dealers' minimised the risks of violence, intimidation and exploitation by unknown organised retail drug distributors and 'gangsters' in clubland. (However, as noted above, we must not assume that all retail drug distributors in clubs are either 'rip off' merchants with poor-quality drugs or unknown to customers.) And thirdly, the collective purchases by friendship networks ahead of the night out resulted in less chance of being caught up in the criminal justice system due to the potentially more risky purchase in clubs where, as we have seen, uniformed and plain-clothes police operate, therefore minimising the risks of being caught up in the reactive, symbolic policing of clubland.

One question which surprised our dance drug sample and involved some extra reassurance of confidentiality in some cases, was asked about half way through the in-depth interview. We asked our dance drug sample from whom they had obtained their drugs that night, explaining that we just wanted to know the form of the relationship – whether it was a friend, a dealer, staff or whoever – rather than exact names and addresses as a few of our respondents at first thought! Of the dance drug sample 53 per cent had procured their drugs from 'friends who regularly get drugs for others', possibly therefore either part of a regular friendship network of three or more people or a retail specialist who the respondent would describe as a friend (see Table 6.1). Another 24 per cent considered they bought their drugs from a 'dealer known to them', presumably a retail specialist working for profit who regularly supplied drugs to the respondent; 17 per cent of the sample obtained their drugs from a 'friend who does not regularly get drugs for others' and therefore was neither a retail specialist nor part of a friendship network that went beyond the two of them. Only 8 per cent of the sample had bought their evening's drugs from a 'dealer unknown to them' and therefore not their regular supplier; 3 per cent had obtained their drugs from family members. Perhaps surprisingly given the observations, interviews and anecdotal evidence of club staff's involvement in the supply of drugs in clubland, no respondents reported obtaining their drugs for the night from pub/club staff, either at the fieldwork club or at any other pub, club or bar.

Table 6.1   Sources of drugs by individual clubs (N = 318)

	Warehouse %	Leisure Centre %	City Centre club %	Total %
Friend: Regularly supplies others	49	53	57	53
Friend: Doesn't regularly supply others	16	17	19	17
Dealer: Known to me	30	23	19	24
Dealer: Unknown to me	10	6	7	8
Staff at any pub, club or bar	0	0	0	0
Work colleagues	1	0	0	0
Family	4	3	2	3
Other	0	3	0	1

These answers show the emphasis placed by young clubbers on building up a relationship through regular contact with a known drugs supplier and also reflect the blurred distinctions between 'dealer' and 'friend': for over half of the dance drug sample their 'dealer' was a friend, or their friend was a 'dealer' depending on one's perspective or which relationship came first. Another quarter had a regular, known 'dealer', although they did not go so far as to call this person a friend. The drugs supply stories provided by our clubbers told of careful organisation and planning to enable them to buy good-quality drugs from a regular 'dealer'/friend well ahead of the big night out, preferably with a group of friends to reduce both the purchase price of the drugs and the time and transport costs of picking up the drugs. Clearly this involved greater legal risks (of possession and possession with intent to supply) for those involved in the transaction, transport and storage of a larger quantity of drugs. The alternative, however, might be considered even riskier in some clubs: buying drugs from distributors in clubs with less chance to check the merchandise before consumption, and a greater chance of being 'ripped off' in some way through poor-quality drugs or theft of money. Or possibly the worse scenario of all from the perspective of some of our clubbers: no retail specialists operating inside the club because of heavy management or policing and the prospect of a drug-free night out.

Trading charities

A third type of drug distribution enterprise identified by Dorn and South, the trading charity, prioritises the drugs experience above the profit motive. Given the size of the tax-free profits available in today's large-scale drugs industry it is perhaps not surprising that trading charities were little in evidence in the commercial dance club scene of our fieldwork period at the end of the 'decade of dance'.

The early days of the underground acid house and 'rave' scene of the late 1980s and early 1990s, discussed in Chapter 2, were characterised by a passion and zeal for both the music and the drugs experience. Ecstasy was a 'new' drug which came to symbolise the early 1990s 'rave' scene in a similar way to the association of LSD with the late 1960s hippie movement, and was taken up with equal enthusiasm. There have been reports of ecstasy evangelists in the early 'rave' scene whose passion for the drug was at least equal to their desire for profit. These were the 'sorters' rather than the 'pushers', those who sorted out a weekend party prescription for their friends and acquaintances and who enjoyed their central position in the dance club scene. This is illustrated in the autobiography of dance entrepreneur and promoter Wayne Anthony (1998). The potential transformative capabilities of ecstasy have been explored by Saunders, at one time considered the British 'godfather' of ecstasy (Saunders, 1993; 1995; 1997) and the role of ecstasy in the development of the British dance club scene has been discussed at length by music journalists, popular commentators and drugs researchers (Wright, 1998; Collin and Godfrey, 1997). Indeed Shapiro describes ecstasy as 'the cultural signifier of a generation' (1999, p. 23).

During the fieldwork period the researchers talked to clubbers who had been involved in the north-west dance scene since the early days of acid house and rave, some of whom had supplied drugs to those they socialised with. Several of these people could be considered trading charities, operating in clubs such as the Hacienda during the vibrancy of the 'Madchester' and 'Flesh' eras, when the celebration of ecstasy, dance music and the communal 'luv'd up' vibe was considered to have been at its peak, before the larger-scale retail specialists had moved into the dance drugs market. One established large-scale dance drugs distributor in both the straight and gay dance clubs of the north-west throughout the whole of the 1990s described his personal transition from trading charity to retail specialist. Profit moved from a secondary motivation, no more than helping fund and facilitate his own clubbing, to a primary motivation as he developed his trade, alongside the move from club-based to home-based sales:

> I finished my degree, the club scene was brilliant, everyone went out, there were nights every day of the week. I had loads of debt but wanted to go out so I got by selling drugs. There was such a wide variety of pills then and you needed to know who to get them off. So people wanted to get them off people they knew. I could get them for this good price. Just get your own night paid for. That was all you were arsed about then.
>
> But then it changed. Your contacts develop. You get a feel for it. If you've got a level head and a bit of quality control. Quality, quality, quality. Quality prevails and people will pay for it. You gravitate round people who sell for quality. You take it yourself. Your reputation and social standing depend on quality, but the profit leads to a nice little lifestyle. Customers are very fickle and it's no different in the drugs trade. People won't complain but they won't come back to you.
>
> As you go deeper it becomes a web of surveillance-avoidance, gangster-avoidance and substance abuse-avoidance. So it's difficult to keep your mental and physical health when leading such a lifestyle. It's a little niche. The need for quality for your own hedonistic pleasure and the use of intelligence to make a life for yourself. Being as discreet as ever. I'm not in it for the notoriety. Most dealers want discretion, not notoriety.
>
> The level of surveillance in the early days was pathetic so you could go around a club with a bag of pills. The police didn't know what to look for or where. You knew the established dealers. There weren't the networks so everyone met in the clubs and bought their drugs there. Now clubs are the front line of detection. Now with years of experience people avoid the front line. Club dealers are younger, it's worse quality, they are into the image, the notoriety. Most people have learnt the social networks and go to people's houses. Less people buy in clubs now because there's more risk. Plus the money's not there. The mark up's not the same. There used to be 100 per cent mark up, buy pills for £8 and sell for £15. It's not worth the risk now. You don't get more than a few quid if that. Buy for £3 and sell for £5 or £6.

Not surprisingly, the repurcussions of such illegality in the purchase and sale of dance drugs for such large numbers of clubbers included some criminal convictions: one in five (20 per cent) of our interview sample (N = 362) reported drug-related cautions or convictions. As we can see from Table 6.2, the north-west dance drug sample underrepresents Class B offences and possession offences in comparison with national statistics for cautions and convictions in 1997 under the 1971 Misuse of Drugs Act. Many of these drug-related offences will have been obtained during routine policing of pubs, clubs and the streets because most clubbers carry their drugs with them at some point between obtaining and consuming them. These indictments will also have been built up over the years that clubbers were drug users, some of whom had considerable repertoires of experimentation from their teens, as we have seen in Chapter 4.

Table 6.2   Comparison of drug-related cautions and convictions with Home Office official statistics

	North-west sample 1998 % (N = 362)	Official statistics* 1998 % (N = 149,907)
Class A	12	19
Class B	44	84
Class C	15	2
Classes A & B combined	16	n/a
Possession	77	90
Trafficking	15	14
Any	20	n/a

* Source: Corkery (2000a).

How were these drugs offenders dealt with in the criminal justice system? For the largest proportion of these clubbers (48 per cent) they received a caution; 15 per cent were fined and 8 per cent were imprisoned, with 8 per cent receiving variations of suspended sentence, probation, community service and combination orders. This is very similar to national Home Office official statistics on drugs offenders for the same year, with 47 per cent of those cautioned, convicted or compounded for drugs offences in 1998 being cautioned, 23 per cent being fined and 8 per cent receiving an immediate custodial sentence (Corkery, 2000a).

If we look at clubbers' concerns regarding the illegality of their drugs consumption, their concerns lay with the policing and regulation of their leisure spaces, rather than with the inherent illegality of their actions or their incidental connections with organised criminals through drug distribution chains. When asked if they perceived their drug use to be problematic in any way regarding the fact that it was illegal, only four of our dance drug sample (1 per cent) said they felt the purchase of illegal drugs was in some way problematic for them. By contrast a third of the sample (33 per cent) felt that the knock-on policing and regulation of clubland was a problem for them. This supports clubbers' concerns about the policing of dance drug use discussed in Chapter 5.

The illegality of widespread leisure-time recreational drug use by young people from a range of social backgrounds in dance club settings has broader implications for these people's lives, however. For one dance drug user 'he considers the illegality of drug use a problem for him because of his intended profession – barrister – and imagines reading the headlines in the Sun' (010108). And even the smallest indication of possible drug use could lead to unexpected contact with the police authorities, as one respondent found out. 'He hasn't suffered many negative experiences through drugs apart from once being strip searched and internally examined at an airport because he had a Rizla packet with a corner torn off' (031103). The ambiguities of such widespread law-breaking by young people from a wide range of backgrounds were apparent to our clubbers, leading one clubber to observe that 'everyone knows what goes on in clubs but still you have to be careful because it is illegal' (210102).

Thus in summary, most clubbers in this study paid for the drugs they consumed, with the organisation of obtaining them shared between friendship groups or bought directly from a drug distributor or 'dealer' known to them or considered to be a friend. Clubbers spoke of a wide range of supply arrangements with a spectrum of roles in the chain of supply and consumption that did not neatly fit the popular 'user versus dealer' dichotomy. Roles varied according to access to finances, access to transport, potential profits, periods of 'drought' in the supply chain and other such issues of access and availability. Clubbers' aims included maximising the chances of purchasing good-quality drugs at the lowest price in time for a big night out, whilst minimising the risks of being caught up in the criminal justice system and arrested, or being intimidated, threatened or 'ripped off' by unscrupulous drugs retail specialists.

Clubbers were not unduly concerned about their illegal transactions and presumably therefore their 'wheeling and dealing' with drug distribution networks. For some of the older, more established clubbers in this study, the attempts over the years to procure drugs and establish contact with drug distributors meant they had built up a degree of experience and confidence in such negotiations. They expressed far more concern about the official responses of the police and club staff which arose out of their criminal behaviour. This finding is supported when we turn our attention to specific incidents of harassment later in the chapter and look at who clubbers reported feeling intimidated by. In contrast to popular and media portrayals of clubland, 'dealers' will feature far less than the police, club staff and even other clubbers.

Playing safe: perceptions of safety and inclusion in clubland

Literary and criminological representations of the city since the urbanisation of nineteenth-century Britain have included images of a dark, seedy, labyrinthine underworld, where aspects of unregulated youth, popular culture, immorality and violence have been linked to the fears of the respectable classes. (For a discussion of representations of the city in criminology and literature see for example Pearson, 1983; Cohen, 1981; Mayhew, 1981; Stedman Jones, 1971.) In the contemporary city, urban youth culture has been discussed in terms of its physical and symbolic location in a deregulated 'wild zone'. Wild zones are located beyond the panopticon of modern regulatory culture, where crime and leisure are linked on a continuum between ordinary consumer culture and deviant play, where speed and movement are prioritised, illustrated in such occurrences as joy riding and computer hacking as well as dance parties and drug use (Stanley, 1997; Rojek, 2000).

Violence and insecurity have traditionally been associated with being outside on the city streets, in the 'public' world, in opposition to the sanctuary and the safety of the home. Feminists have challenged these notions since the 1970s, and the work of rape crisis and refuge centres, feminist sociologists, and criminologists conducting victimisation studies have shown that violence and insecurity are also located within the 'private' sphere of the home for both adults and children (e.g. Hanmer et al., 1989). Definitions of violence have expanded to include more than just physical violence, but also sexual, emotional, psychological, economic and non-physical abuse and exploitation. Indeed it has been argued that 'there are no single, uniform or even clear meanings of violence' (Phoenix, 1999, p. 263). In this section we will consider our clubbers' perceptions of safety and security, located in the challenge to the public/private dichotomy of fear/safety.

Given that household victimisation studies such as the British Crime Survey show a statistically significant relationship between experiences of violence and being 'out and about' on the streets and in pubs and clubs, we might expect our sociable sample of young adults to be aware of and experience high levels of violence and intimidation in the course of their clubbing activities (Mirrlees-Black et al., 1998; Tseloni, 1995). Clearly they do experience violence and intimidation on the city streets in and around pubs and clubs. When asked what, if anything, concerned our interview respondents about their safety when going out to clubs, about half of the respondents (53 per cent) voiced concerns. The five main safety concerns for clubbers who expressed specific concerns were physical aggression and violence (25 per cent), issues relating to other people's drinking or drunkenness (19 per cent), verbal aggression and bad 'attitude' of others (15 per cent), and concerns about being stranded and unable to get home (13 per cent). In part this may have been due to previous personal experiences: later in our interview when we asked respondents whether they had ever had problems getting home from clubs, nearly a quarter had (24 per cent).

The issue of safe places is particularly relevant to the ways in which safety in club spaces is mediated by gender, race, socio-economic class, disability and sexual orientation, as we saw in Chapter 2. Massey discusses, in relation to gender in particular, the ways in which:

... space and place, spaces and places, and our senses of them ... are gendered through and through. Moreover they are gendered in a myriad different ways, which vary between cultures and over time. And this gendering of space and place both reflects *and has effects back on* the ways in which gender is constructed and understood in the societies in which we live. (1994, p. 186)

As noted in Chapter 2, issues of gender and safety in clubland have been directly linked to the consumption of alcohol and drugs. The lack of alcohol-related sexual harassment for women and alcohol-related physical aggression for men have been seen as factors which made clubbers in dance clubs feel safer than in traditional night clubs. Perceptions of safety therefore related to lack of alcohol-related hassles for many of our respondents, such as the non-drug user who felt 'far more safe in a club where people are on drugs. I feel alcohol use is far more dangerous and disruptive than drugs' (020201). This was echoed by other female clubbers such as the woman who 'does think that "drug" clubs are nicer places to be than "alcohol" clubs because of the good atmosphere and the lack of aggression' (010105). Similarly one interviewer commented:

She made a big point of saying that in most other clubs she gets groped by men. She reminded me of other female interviewees at the Leisure Centre who are in their thirties and go to clubs which they believe are safe from 'dodgy' men who are intoxicated with alcohol. (160720)

And young men too, the most victimised group in relation to self-reported violence in victimisation studies (Mirrlees-Black et al., 1998), discussed feeling safer in dance clubs than in pubs and night clubs where immoderate alcohol consumption was a key feature of the night out for the majority of customers. One respondent said 'he'd never had any trouble in a drugs club but in others with "pissed up people" he'd had to talk his way out of trouble on four occasions' (070809). Another respondent said the thing which concerned him about clubs was 'getting into fights. Not bad at dance clubs. Townie clubs are more scary than dance clubs, different clientele. At dance clubs they're more into music than just getting pissed. That's the way I find it' (030201). For a third respondent, 'he dislikes clubs when there are "drunken yobs looking for a fight"' (100403). And we even interviewed one man who admitted to being one of those 'drunken yobs': 'my relationships are generally better with people because when I'm on the beer I start fighting' (140711).

This view was shared by non-drug users as well as drug users. One non-user who illustrates the widespread tolerance of dance drug use by non-using clubbers, said regarding dance drug use:

It doesn't bother me. I don't worry about the legality or their health, they're old enough to look after themselves. The people on the drugs don't cause the problems. It's the people on alcohol. I know it's a cliché but that's my experience. (150205)

Dance clubs were not always the model of perfectly antisexist, egalitarian and tolerant behaviour, however. One female clubber pointed out that she 'felt very safe in clubs or at least in the Warehouse club, although I have been touched up by a "creepy man" in there once' (011102).

For gay and lesbian clubbers specific experiences of violence and harassment in dance venues and on the city streets resulted in some respondents commenting on the greater sense of safety in gay/lesbian and mixed dance clubs than in straight dance clubs. Truman (forthcoming) has noted, however, that the sense of safety experienced in the geographically distinct gay and lesbian city-centre leisure spaces may be a contingent safety by comparison with a local mixed neighbourhood which may provide a greater ontological security for lesbians. That the gay and lesbian clubbers in our study reported feeling slightly safer in clubland than straight clubbers (see Table 6.3) may be a consequence, at least in part, of interviewing gay and lesbian clubbers in the gay/mixed City Centre club. One gay man said he was 'conscious of dodgy people whatever I'm on but I do feel safer in gay clubs' (170205). For another:

The one thing he was most worried about was 'gay bashing' which had happened to him three times. ... he went to an all-night club in a nearby town ... a lot of young men were standing outside. They hurled abuse at him: 'shit stabber' and 'shirt lifter'. He was very frightened. (200510)

And at the extreme end of sexual violence one man reported having been 'gang-raped back in January and he uses the drugs to forget about it' (180301).

Clubbers also made links between feeling unsafe and the consumption of drugs. Firstly, clubbers discussed their increased vulnerability to physical aggression and violence when intoxicated in clubs. One interviewer noted that his respondent:

Feels unsafe because of the police and clubland's associated 'underworld nastiness', and the fact that he loses his inhibitions totally when intoxicated on drugs or alcohol and is prepared to 'take anyone on' and therefore exposes himself to danger. (151013)

Secondly, clubbers made links between feeling unsafe and taking health-related risks through dance drug consumption in clubs. One interviewer noted that when he asked a respondent about his concerns about his future health and well being 'he doesn't think about the future and said he was "not bothered,

I'm enjoying myself now". But when asked about what concerns him about his safety he said "passing out and dying"' (091107).

By and large, however, the interesting point is that for the clubbers in our sample, they felt safe and secure in clubland. When asked how safe they usually feel when they go out to clubs, that is both in clubs and on journeys to and from clubs, our interview sample (N = 362) in a range from 1 (very unsafe) to 5 (very safe) scored on average 4.26, with a mode of 5. In other words, eight in ten clubbers felt either safe or very safe in and around clubs. There were surprisingly few variations in this feeling of safety between clubbers from different socio-demographic groups and between clubs, as Table 6.3 shows. It is interesting to note, however, that abstainers and drug users felt slightly safer than drinkers in and around clubland, and those driving themselves or being driven home felt slightly safer than those having to rely on public or private hire forms of transport.

Table 6.3   Perceptions of safety (N = 362)

	Mean	Standard Deviation
Female	4.23	0.84
Male	4.28	0.81
White	4.26	0.82
Asian	4.20	0.45
Black	4.20	1.30
Gay/Lesbian	4.40	0.87
Straight	4.23	0.80
Bisexual	4.19	0.87
Abstainer	4.43	0.79
Mainly drugs	4.29	0.78
Half & half	4.28	0.81
Mainly drinking	4.06	0.86
Warehouse	4.20	0.85
Leisure Centre	4.25	0.75
City Centre Club	4.32	0.87
Drive yourself	4.37	0.71
Driven by friend	4.26	0.82
Taxi	4.21	0.88
Bus	4.13	0.83
Overall Mean	4.26	0.82

For many of those interviewed, dance clubs were places with familiar faces, familiar music, familiar expectations and obligations, rules and regulations, experiences and pleasures, that they chose to go to. They were both fun places and safe spaces. Their homes might also provide this sense of well being and familiarity, but for many young people for whatever reasons, of whatever race, gender, sexual orientation, socio-economic background or family situation, home might not necessarily be associated with comfort, safety or security. And for young people stopped on the streets by the police, living in cramped conditions in parents' houses, facing possible attack, harassment, hate crimes or homophobia in day-to-day life, the club might provide a sense of belonging, acceptance, tolerance; that feeling of being 'at home' articulated by our clubbers. In this way pubs, clubs and bars might represent safety in contrast to work, domestic worlds, families, the streets and the routes between bars and clubs. As Thornton has pointed out, whilst for American post-war young adults the car has represented their own social space away from family and adults, for British young people the club is more likely to be the physical and symbolic space owned by young people (1995). This notion of the club as freedom, security and 'home' is reflected in comments by the following clubbers when asked what they liked about going clubbing. For example, 'the freedom to be myself. No one in the club knows who I am and I can share my personality characteristics with them' (210102). A second clubber explained that 'going to clubs really boosts your social life and I feel really *at home* when out clubbing. "It's really me"' (010708). A third clubber also offered up the analogy with home: 'It's a lifestyle. It feels like home. I do drugs naturally, all my friends take drugs. I love my lifestyle' (090513). 'Clubs are a different world, a change to normal life' (010803).

Our sample by definition is those who have been included in clubland – they have self-selected and been selected to enter the club on the fieldwork night – but it is a conditional inclusion in clubland. Such conditional inclusion depends on socio-economic background, race, gender and sexual orientation with the distinct socio-demographics of club culture discussed in Chapter 2. Conditional inclusion is also determined by taste, appearance, clothing, 'attitude', indeed the hipness which Thornton terms 'subcultural capital' (1995, p. 11). This means that whilst clubs might feel like home to some of the clubbers we interviewed, others will not have made it past the front door or will have remained on the periphery even once inside.

There was conditional inclusion of 'straights' or heterosexual clubbers into the City Centre club at weekends, for example, with door staff following informal guidelines for inclusion and exclusion on Fridays and Saturdays where the specified door policy was 'gays/lesbians and straight friends'. Such conditional inclusion was not based on direct questions about sexual orientation, current relationships, sexual practices or friendship networks because these questions were deemed unacceptable and discriminatory by door staff. Instead inclusion depended on the acquisition of 'gay' cultural knowledge relating to pubs, clubs and magazines, alongside critical assessments of clubbers' appearance by staff. As Skeggs notes, 'appearance is a crucial aspect of criminalizing and entry or not into public space' (2000, p. 130). (For further discussion on safety, space

and sexuality see also Moran, 2000, and Whittle, 1994.) One of the male door
staff at the City Centre club summed up this attitude to vetting clubbers:

> If a group arrive at the door there has to be more gay people than straight
> people, I won't let any groups of straight people come in. I ask what clubs
> they go to and what magazines they read. Customers are never asked directly
> about their sexuality as that is seen as an invasion of people's privacy. In the
> end, though, you can just tell. (200510)

Experiences of safety and well being on a club night out can also be broadened
to include the provision of a physically safe environment inside clubs. The need
for clubs with well-ventilated rooms, monitoring of air quality, air temperature
and air humidity, a layout designed to cope with capacity crowds, 'chill out'
areas away from the music with adequate seating facilities, access to free drinking
water, on-site drugs outreach workers and first-aid staff, licensed and trained
security staff, and so on have been well documented elsewhere (Newcombe,
1994; Saunders, 1995). The cavernous arenas at the Leisure Centre, with high
ceilings and plenty of space, meant high room temperatures were not a problem.
Two of our three fieldwork clubs, however, became very hot on summer evenings
as capacity peaked in the last few hours of weekend club nights. These two clubs
both had the possibility of opening various external doors to cool off overheated
clubbers but door staff insisted on keeping the doors closed in line with fire
safety regulations and made a point of closing doors when clubbers opened
them. At the Warehouse the central courtyard allowed customers to leave the
club to cool down at the tables and benches provided, if also prepared to leave
the music and atmosphere, but at the City Centre club there was no access to
the open air.

In summary, half of clubbers were in some way concerned about their safety
in and around clubland, with particular concerns about physical and verbal
aggression, other people's drunkenness and problems getting home at the end
of the night. Distinctions in perceptions of safety were made between different
clubs: night clubs versus dance clubs, straight clubs versus gay clubs, and as we
shall see later in this chapter, northern versus southern clubs. Nevertheless, eight
in ten clubbers felt safe or very safe in clubland and many discussed clubs with
specific reference to feeling safe and 'at home' by comparison with work, their
domestic lives, or out and about on the streets. This suggests the need to modify
popular and media portrayals of late 1990s/millennial clubland and the surrounding city streets as excessively dangerous, full of 'gangsters', guns and
'dodgy' drugs. (As we discussed in Chapter 5, even the quality and purity of the
illicit dance drugs consumed by clubbers appeared from our in-club urine samples
to be of generally higher quality than we, the laboratory staff or the clubbers
themselves expected.) Clubbers discussed clubs in terms of them being their

play space, their fun place, and perhaps most surprisingly, for many young adults clubs were also their safe place. However, the conditional nature of inclusion in clubland means that the attitude and behaviour of others could infringe on this pleasure space, as we shall discuss in more detail in the next section.

Experiences of violence, intimidation and regulation

We turn our attention now from perceptions of safety and security to experiences of violence and harassment. We asked our interview sample whether they had ever been hassled or felt intimidated, either inside or outside a club, by five different categories of people they regularly came into contact with in clubland: other clubbers, club staff, drug 'dealers', police operating inside clubs and police operating outside clubs (see Table 6.4).

Table 6.4   Experiences of intimidation (N = 357)

	Warehouse %	Leisure Centre %	City Centre %	Total %
Other clubbers	55	44	54	51
Club staff	45	45	38	43
Drug 'dealers'	21	9	11	14*
Police inside	7	7	12	9
Police outside	20	27	12	20*

* p < 0.5

Other clubbers

Half of all interview respondents said they had been hassled or felt intimidated at some time by other clubbers. For those who felt intimidated there were four main categories of concern: 36 per cent specified verbal aggression or bad 'attitude', 24 per cent reported sexual harassment, 18 per cent specified physical aggression or violence and 15 per cent discussed issues related to other people's drinking or drunkenness. Many of these incidents of harassment and intimidation were linked to more general male aggression and the 'machismo' of young men in British licensed leisure contexts (Marsh and Fox Kibby, 1992; Collison, 1996; Tomsen, 1997). Typical anecdotes included fighting between local factions such as 'Newtown boys wanting fights' (071117). There were also accounts of altercations between men over women. One respondent reported he had been 'talking to a girl who had a boyfriend who hit me with a piece of wood and I had to go to hospital. Had to have stitches in my head' (010206).

Club staff

Over four in ten of those interviewed had felt intimidated or hassled by club staff and when asked to specify which staff in particular, nearly two-thirds of those (64 per cent) said 'bouncers' or security/door staff, 10 per cent said club staff in general and only 2 per cent specified bar staff. Although the form that this harassment or intimidation took was mainly verbal aggression or bad 'attitude' (63 per cent), of concern was the reporting of excessive searches and strip searches for over a fifth (21 per cent) of those who reported feeling intimidated by club staff, and also the experiences of physical aggression or violence for nearly a tenth (9 per cent) of those reporting feeling intimidated. Typical of the comments we received about door staff were experiences of having 'felt intimidated by bouncers in general' (010405). These incidents and experiences were reported by female as well as male clubbers. One young woman told the interviewer that 'in the City Centre club my friend was "touched up" by the bouncer. We complained, were punched and thrown out' (030612).

Searches by security/door staff was a subject which animated many of those we interviewed. This is not surprising given the relative power and centrality of security/door staff to life in the club. They have the power to include or exclude clubbers from their club, they can forcibly eject those already inside the club, search and detain customers, hand them over to the police and in each of these operations can make customers feel humiliated in front of their friends and peers (Marsh and Fox Kibby, 1992; Morris, 1998). Door staff would not necessarily agree with this analysis of their relative power in clubs by comparison with clubbers, however. One of the door staff at the Leisure Centre discussed how restricted at work he felt by the law:

> If you jump in to stop a fight and do too much damage you could face an ABH or GBH charge. And the police wouldn't back you up. If a door man is hurt he'd probably just get a PC and a couple of Special Constables round. If there's a clubber hurt you'd get vans, dogs, everything. The cards are stacked against door staff.

Many clubbers' comments related to zealous searches and surveillance by security/door staff. Although there may have been some exaggeration in these details of excessive searching and aggression, the frequency of such anecdotes about the fieldwork sites and other clubs implies that there were serious problems with the working practices of security staff and the boundaries of their methods of regulation. For example one respondent reported that a 'bouncer at a London club made me strip to pants outside in winter, wearing only shoes' (010209) One interviewer noted clubbers' comments on being strip searched by door staff at the Leisure Centre:

> Two of my interviewees mentioned about illegal strip searches done at the Leisure Centre, which I had heard about before from an interviewee at the Warehouse club. This was both males and females, who I was told if they

refused were thrown out. And there was mention of beatings after strip searching. This I find very shocking as an abuse of power, particularly as the crowd are generally young. (090513)

Respondents' reports, confirmed by co-ordinators' observations, included details of strip searches at other dance events, sometimes down to clubbers' underwear, being asked to take shoes and socks off, and sometimes being handed over to police called to the club or waiting outside the venue in a van for that purpose. The co-ordinators witnessed security staff in male and female toilets in dance clubs other than the three fieldwork sites standing on toilet seats and looking over cubicle partitions to check customers using toilets were not consuming drugs within the cubicle. Toilet cubicles not infrequently had their locks removed to assist in this surveillance of customers. This led to resentment by many of the clubbers we interviewed who felt that too many dance club promoters and venue management and staff wanted to 'have their cake and eat it': to obtain the profits and employment from all-night dance events and yet unrealistically and zealously police several hundred or several thousand people dancing for up to 12 hours in an attempt to stop them taking stimulant drugs. Even the door staff recognised and reflected on this dilemma. The balance between efficient club security and the facilitation of a good club night was discussed by one of the door staff at the Leisure Centre in relation to his perspective on door policy and the issue of the sale and consumption of drugs:

> It's a balance between not letting people deal and take drugs openly, taking the piss out of the door staff on the one hand. And on the other, to accept that people are here to have a good time, dance and take drugs. And if they weren't here we wouldn't have a job.

Such comprehensive searches led clubbers firstly, to more creative methods of hiding drugs such as inside their underwear or in one case taped to genitals! 'He mentioned one incident at Helter Skelter [large-scale hardcore dance event] during which they searched him five times but found nothing because they were sellotaped to his penis' (101040).

Secondly, stringent searches encouraged the consumption of drugs before entry to the club. Clubbers tended to consume their drugs before entry to a club if the club was known for either particularly zealous searches or a strict policy of passing clubbers to the police if found to be in possession of drugs for personal use. This practice raises health concerns for clubbers because it encouraged the pre-club simultaneous consumption of larger quantities of different drugs by our poly-drug using clubbers. (This is particularly worrying in the case of all-night dance events such as occured at the Warehouse club because a considerable quantity of drugs might be consumed at one sitting rather than staggered or 'stacked' throughout the night.) Harm minimisation advice for dance drug use, familiar to many users and targeted particularly at women, includes the suggestion that drugs are consumed in small quantities across the course of a whole night out rather than at one sitting (Scottish Drugs Forum, 1996).

The relative position of power of security/door staff in relation to entry and removal of clubbers from clubs, maintaining order, and controlling drug distribution and organised crime, points to the need for training, regulation, licensing and accountability. The concerns and problems expressed by clubbers in this study add weight to this call. Moves in some cities towards door staff schemes employing only licensed, fully trained door staff are thus clearly welcome. However, the tensions between promoting organised dance events and policing the dance drug use which occurs at them, expressed by door staff themselves, need to be directly addressed.

Drug 'dealers'

It is interesting to note that by comparison with over four in ten clubbers feeling intimidated by club staff and half intimidated by other clubbers, only 49 of our interview respondents (14 per cent) felt harassed by drug 'dealers' either inside or outside a club. There were considerable variations between clubs in this, with respondents being significantly more likely to report such intimidation at the Warehouse club. For nearly half of those who reported intimidation by drug 'dealers' at the three clubs, (21, 43 per cent) the harassment took the form of verbal aggression or bad 'attitude', for 19 (39 per cent) it related to the drug deal itself (quality issues, exploitation, being 'ripped off'), and for five respondents (10 per cent) the concerns related to the interview respondents identifying *themselves* as drug 'dealers' and having problems with other drug distributors in clubs. Only four respondents out of the 362 we interviewed mentioned the use or threatened use of weapons such as knives, guns, syringes and CS 'tear' gas.

It has been noted in other research studies of young people's leisure that trouble is often associated with 'others' and 'elsewhere' (Measham, 2000). Our clubbers also located trouble elsewhere, both geographically and temporally, as illustrated by the following quotes. Trouble was located 'elsewhere' such as in London clubs:

> He and his friends had just left a club in Brixton when someone appeared to speak from behind. He looked round and a man had a gun pointing at him. He asked if he had any cocaine on him and when he was told no, the gunman said words to the effect of 'oh never mind' and simply walked away. (050612)

A second respondent had been to a 'London club – full of drug dealers – went to dance where one dealer pulled a gun out' (010209).

And trouble was also located in the past, usually a non-specific time period of a few years ago. One male clubber said 'he's been hassled by drug dealers before in a club. That was a long time ago at another club, where they used to pull out machetes and say "buy your drugs off me"' (030703).

We can see, therefore, that whilst the single biggest perceived threat to clubbers' safety came from other clubbers, three times more clubbers felt threatened by club staff than by drug 'dealers'. Only four respondents reported ever having felt threatened by 'dealers' armed with weapons. This is in stark contrast to portrayals by some elements of the media, the police and club management of omniscient/omnipotent organised criminals, the 'gangsters' with guns, which characterised the discourse of dance and the closure of dance clubs in the late 1990s (e.g. Swanton, 1998). By contrast, clubbers were rather more 'concerned about the danger that "pissheads" and "plastic gangsters" pose' (081119).

Police inside clubs

Under one in ten clubbers interviewed (31, 9 per cent) reported having been intimidated or harassed by the police inside clubs. The four main types of intimidation were verbal aggression or bad 'attitude' (nine respondents), being questioned by the police (seven respondents), the police 'raiding' or shutting down a club which they were attending (five respondents) and harassment by undercover police (five respondents).

More generally, a third (31 per cent) of interview respondents felt that the police had affected their night out by their actions in some way. Of these respondents, 35 per cent felt that the atmosphere in the club had been spoilt by the police walking around, 23 per cent had been caught up in a police raid of a club, and 19 per cent had more significant contact with the police in clubland, either personally having been searched or arrested, or having friends who were searched or arrested by the police. Yet all of this was tolerated and accepted, and of course counteracted.

One might think that those not taking drugs had nothing to fear from the police presence inside clubs, but for our non-drug using respondents the police presence was off-putting enough to make them consider cancelling their planned evening out clubbing. One non-drug user who discovered a police raid in action as he was about to enter a club saw a 'big search for drugs in a club so we didn't go in. Too much. We saw the police in the van so we didn't go in even though we weren't doing drugs ourselves' (010206).

Whilst police raids on clubs may be aimed at netting the organised criminals and drugs retail specialists, there was anecdotal evidence that 'ordinary' clubbers could also get caught up in police activities. Staff at the Warehouse club, for example, said 'there was a police raid in the club a while ago and when they didn't find the big fish they'd hoped to get they ended up arresting a couple of lads for smoking a joint'.

The City Centre club was also subject to police operations inside the club although not the dramatic Tactical Aid midnight march through the club that occurred every week in the Warehouse club. We noted:

> It appears plain clothes were in operation tonight. Members of our research team were standing in the foyer interviewing and said the police were coming in and grabbing individuals and taking them outside for questioning. Talking to one of our interviewers, a man said it happens nearly every week and that the week before he'd been taken out and strip searched in the van before being let back inside. (Co-ordinator's fieldwork notes)

Police attendance at British dance clubs directly affects clubbers, with one in ten reporting having felt hassled or intimidated by police in clubs in some way. Moreover, police operations in clubland led to a third of clubbers reporting that the police had negatively affected their night out in some way. However, it was clubbers' contact with the police outside the club space which caused them greater concern, as discussed in the following section.

Police outside clubs

Almost twice as many clubbers interviewed felt cause for concern about the police outside clubs compared with inside clubs (see Table 6.4). A fifth of interview respondents reported feeling harassed or intimidated by police outside clubs, with over a quarter of these (28 per cent) saying their main concern was being searched or strip searched by the police, whereas for 21 per cent it related to the general police presence on the streets, and for 18 per cent it related to verbal aggression or a perceived bad 'attitude' by the police. Interestingly, harassment or intimidation by the police outside clubs, on the streets and elsewhere, was significantly related to which clubs our respondents were interviewed in. Those clubbers interviewed at the Leisure Centre, with a younger, more working-class customer base, were most likely to report harassment whereas those clubbers interviewed at the City Centre club with an older, more professional and mixed/gay customer base were least likely to report such harassment.

Respondents reported incidents of being pulling out of clubs or club queues and searched in police vans waiting nearby, adding further incentive for clubbers to consume their night's drugs before entering clubs. Again the potential consequences will include firstly, some people consuming their night's drugs supply in one large dose rather than smaller amounts spread out across the course of the evening, a preferable harm minimisation strategy. And secondly, others might carefully conceal drugs on their person before entry, depending on the comprehensiveness of searches at entry into the club and the level of surveillance once inside the club.

There were cat and mouse tales of police interactions with clubbers, sometimes related to the suspected possession of drugs:

> He was once arrested for suspected possession. He had some cocaine in his sock and when he was arrested they put him in the police van and drove around quite wildly. He said the police did this to 'shake him up'. During this rough ride he was able to discreetly take the cocaine out of his sock and put it into the wheel well in the back of the van. They then strip searched him but he had nothing on him. (040104)

Sometimes it was related to the movement of clubbers en masse to and from dance venues. 'Outside the club no one would move from the car park after the club so they brought in the police and they let off tear gas and the fire brigade used hoses to get everyone to move' (090703). And sometimes these cat and mouse tales were a part of broader police contact with the respondent's family and community, as illustrated by this Leisure Centre clubber:

> The police became a major theme in the interview. He has had many encounters with the police over the years. One cop has an old rivalry with his father from their school days and he feels he takes his hatred of his father out on him. He gets pulled by the police up to four times a week just because he is known rather than because of his behaviour. (141105)

As we have seen, the people we interviewed felt surprisingly safe in clubs, although they did experience bad 'attitude' from some other clubbers on an occasional basis, from security/door staff, the police and to a lesser extent from 'dealers'. Police and club management and staff made clear their perceived distinctions between 'genuine' clubbers and 'dealers'. Police and club management expressed their concerns about trying to control the behaviour of organised criminals and protecting 'genuine' clubbers from these so-called 'gangsters' and 'dealers'. Clubbers, by contrast, did not make such clear distinctions between clubbers and 'dealers', rather their concerns related to the police and club staff themselves. Negative experiences were reported particularly surrounding excessive personal searches and surveillance of clubbers by police on the streets and by door staff at clubs. But once clubbers proceeded past the police street patrols and past possibly erratic and over-zealous door staff, they felt able to relax and enjoy the atmosphere inside the club space. It was an obstacle course which clubbers seemed to feel was well worth running.

Clubland at the crossroads: transport issues

Closely related to issues of safety and security is the question of transport to and from clubs wherever they might be located. Our three clubs illustrate three different transport dilemmas for clubbers. The Warehouse club was located outside the central hub of the city nightlife, shopping and finance districts down a back street in a derelict inner-city area surrounded by dark streets, disused warehouses, half-demolished office blocks, condemned buildings and empty lots awaiting redevelopment. With public transport in the city centre more than a 15-minute walk away, clubbers relied on taxis, private cars or a rather uninviting walk to and from the club down poorly lit streets past a known back-street 'red light' area. There was a very small car park nearby but it was not considered to be a safe enough neighbourhood to leave cars unattended. The City Centre club, by comparison, was on a busy, well-lit main road with other pubs, clubs and bars nearby and was well served by the buses, trains and taxi ranks of the city centre. Its central location also allowed the possibility of walking and cycling home. The main problems for clubbers attending the City Centre club related to tensions over parking spaces and taxis in front of the club. However, with bus stops for night buses which served key residential areas only a few minutes' walk away from the club, for those without enough money, forward planning or energy to acquire taxis, staggering on to the nearby night bus was a possibility for many customers, the main deterrents being the weather and the wait. The Leisure Centre was located several miles outside a city centre and with a very large car park but no public transport links at all. Therefore most clubbers were obliged to use private cars to get to and from the dance event. There was a handful of organised coach tours, minibuses and taxis but the distance from the Leisure Centre to most residential areas and the considerable distance travelled to the club by many of the regulars meant taxis were beyond most clubbers' means except for those who lived locally.

When we looked at how clubbers planned to return home from the club on the fieldwork night, nearly half of our interview sample of clubbers (47 per cent) planned to return home by private car: 28 per cent had a friend driving them home and 19 per cent planned to drive themselves home (see Table 6.5). A further 40 per cent planned to take a taxi home. Only 6 per cent planned to return home using some sort of public or hired transport: bus, train or coach; 3 per cent planned to walk and less than 1 per cent planned to cycle.

Clearly transport is a key issue for clubland with hundreds of thousands of clubbers – in varying degrees of intoxication, in club clothes often not particularly practical for outdoor wear, with considerable amounts of cash and credit cards in their pockets and purses (as we have seen earlier in this chapter) – needing to get safely to and from venues. City centres allow some limited degree of public transport and taxi hire, finances permitting. Hence 66 per cent of customers at the Warehouse club and 45 per cent of customers at the City Centre club planned to take a taxi and one-fifth of customers at both of these clubs planned to use some form of public or 'alternative' transport. A minority (33 per cent at the City Centre club and 21 per cent at the Warehouse club) planned to use private cars to get home. But for out-of-town dance venues, in part granted licence approval because of their location well away from residential areas, public transport links are very limited. Given both the wide catchment area and as we have seen, the lower socio-economic customer base at hardcore dance events often held in these leisure centres, taxis are not feasible for most clubbers, therefore elevating the importance of cars to clubbers. Hence the sharp contrast between the Leisure Centre and the other two clubs regarding modes of transport. Nine in ten Leisure Centre customers planned to get home by car whilst only one in ten planned to use a taxi, with very few other modes of transport mentioned.

Table 6.5   Methods of transport home from clubs (N = 354)

	Warehouse %	Leisure Centre %	City Centre %	Mean distance home km	Standard Deviation	Total %
Taxi	66	10	45	54	99	40
Driven by friend	14	52	18	46	37	28
Drive yourself	7	36	15	50	64	19
Bus	7	1	6	41	56	4
Walk	1	0	8	7	13	3
Train	2	0	2	54	33	1
Cycle	0	0	3	54	39	1
Coach	0	0	1	83	–	0
Other	3	1	3	99	77	2
Total	100	100	100	50	74	100

It serves as an interesting illustration of the limitations of transport options experienced by clubbers that the research team, too, felt so frustrated that they also resorted to driving themselves to and from work, despite plans to provide taxis for them:

> Craig drove us to work last night, we're all so sick of waiting for taxis at the end of the night, it's a real downer. Dean got the bus, four of us went home with Craig, leaving just Debbie and Lucy to get a taxi home. Debbie was so pissed off with taxis she decided to drive to work tonight, as did various others so we won't need any taxis home afterwards. (Co-ordinator's fieldwork notes)

However, whilst the researchers saw transport as problematic, in fact under a quarter (24 per cent) of our interview sample reported ever having had problems getting home safely from clubs, quite low considering they lived a mean distance of 50 kilometres from the club in which they were interviewed on the fieldwork night. However, for the quarter of those experiencing problems getting home safely, a quarter of these (22, 26 per cent) had experienced taxi problems of one sort or another. The importance of obtaining a taxi home at the end of the club night meant that clubbers sometimes faced tensions with other clubbers over taxis in short supply, or risked their own personal safety by hailing private-hire taxis on the streets, or even unlicensed private cars driven by members of the general public hoping to earn extra income. Increasing ownership of mobile phones by young people meant that access to telephones to call taxi companies was no longer the main problem in obtaining private-hire taxis, rather the difficulty lay in clubbers trying to make direct contact with taxi controllers at busy times with phone lines frequently engaged, or controllers trying to make contact with their drivers. This problem was particularly acute at the Warehouse club, outside the hub of the city centre public transport routes and taxi ranks, with two-thirds of its clubbers all wanting to go home by taxi at more or less the same time, as noted by the co-ordinator during the course of the fieldwork:

> Lots of private-hire taxis go past the Warehouse club during the evening and pick up 'casual' passengers, although they're not supposed to do that. In fact it's difficult to phone for a taxi and get a private-hire cab the legitimate way – as we are finding out for ourselves at the end of our night's work – because controllers said the drivers switch off their radios and cruise the streets hoping to pick up a casual fare and don't call in to the controller. (Co-ordinator's fieldwork notes)

The acquisition of taxis could also be problematic at the City Centre club, including for the research team:

> Disaster getting home after fieldwork last night. Both taxis were very late, it was pouring with rain and we had to wait outside the club for over half an hour. Some researchers who'd been waiting for the first of the two taxis had to wait an hour. Jon and I didn't have coats, none of us had umbrellas and we all got soaked. We rang the taxi firm several times and they kept saying it'll be two minutes. We were not amused. We all wanted to go home to bed. The researchers had worked hard last night from 10pm to 2.30am without much of a break. (Co-ordinator's fieldwork notes)

Looking further at those who had experienced problems getting home safely, a quarter (22, 26 per cent) had transport-related problems other than taxis, such as missing public transport or breaking down in a car; 16 respondents (19 per cent) had been lost or stranded somewhere after clubbing. Only four respondents (5 per cent) reported ever having been involved in a vehicle crash after clubbing. One might conclude, therefore, that although inadvisable for nearly half of clubbers to be returning home by private car and probably having about an hour's drive ahead of them, it appears that they have strategies to minimise the harm resulting to themselves and others from this possible further risk-taking behaviour at the end of their night out.

Whilst the location of clubs, the timing of closure and hence the lack of available or affordable public transport alternatives meant many clubbers felt they had no choice but to drive home after a night out, clubbers discussed their harm minimisation strategies in relation to driving home. These strategies may in part explain the low levels of reported motor accidents and a couple of these will be discussed below.

Firstly, we turn our attention to the unnamed, unknown friends who were driving people home on the fieldwork night. Of the 47 per cent of our interview sample who reported returning home by private car, six in ten (101, 59 per cent) were being driven by friends and only four in ten were driving themselves. Thus three in ten clubbers had a friend driving them home. What we do not know from our data is whether the friends who planned to drive home these clubbers were drinking or taking drugs on the fieldwork night. It is evident from interviews, conversations and observations that some of these driver friends were under the influence of alcohol and/or illicit drugs. It may have been that those who were neither drinking nor taking drugs on the fieldwork night (5 per cent of our club sweep sample) were amongst the friends driving people home. Although we cannot be sure how many of the nominated drivers were abstainers, we can see how many of the abstainers we interviewed were nominated drivers. Table 6.6 shows that over half of those abstaining from alcohol and dance drugs on the fieldwork night (57 per cent) drove themselves and others home at the end of the night. We noticed a degree of expectation, even obligation for abstainers to drive the rest of the group home after their night out. This led to expressions of irritation and resentment amongst some abstainers, particularly the young women at the Leisure Centre, that they were expected to drive home their boyfriends and friends at the end of the night because 'drug free', even though they might be tired from their dancing exertions, perhaps even more tired than their drug-using friends who were under the influence of stimulant drugs.

Secondly, we can find out a little more about the fifth of clubbers who reported driving themselves home after the club. Table 6.6 shows that only about one in 20 of those who were drinking (with or without drugs) on the fieldwork night planned to drive themselves home after the club whereas one in three of those we interviewed who considered themselves to be mainly taking drugs planned to drive themselves home afterwards. This suggests that clubbers are more reluctant to drink and drive than consume drugs and drive. However, given that four times more drinkers had friends driving them home than reported driving themselves home, we may have uncovered a greater reluctance to report drinking and driving than to report drug use and driving because of the growing consensus against drinking and driving.

Table 6.6   **Methods of transport home from clubs by drink/drug status (N = 351)**

	Mainly drinking %	Mainly Drugs %	Half & half %	Abstainer %	Total %
Taxi	65	24	52	14	40
Driven by friend	19	32	25	29	27
Drive yourself	5	35	6	57	20
Bus	7	2	7	0	5
Walk	2	3	4	0	3
Train	2	1	2	0	1
Cycle	0	1	1	0	1
Coach	0	1	0	0	0
Other	0	3	3	0	2
Total	100	100	100	100	100

Whilst not excusing driving under the possible influence of legal or illegal drugs, we should also note that some drivers discussed the care they took in order to drive home as safely as possible in the circumstances. Their harm minimisation strategies included consuming alcohol and illicit drugs at the earliest opportunity in their evening out, in the certainty of dancing vigorously for up to six or eight hours. They therefore attempted to postpone their drive home until the effects of the legal and illicit drugs they had consumed were waning. For example, amphetamine lasts up to eight hours depending on the dose, the full effects of ecstasy last three to four hours, cocaine lasts for about half an hour and poppers last for a minute or two (Saunders, 1995). This suggests that amphetamine will be of greatest concern in relation to clubbers driving under the influence of dance drugs after a night out, along with cannabis which is used in a variety of locations before and after clubbing.

Two problems arise with clubbers' attempts to delay their drive home until the decline in the effects of drugs consumption. Firstly, these 'guestimates' were flawed by the unknown aspects of consuming illegally manufactured street drugs of variable quality. Secondly, given the amounts of alcohol and drugs consumed by drivers on the fieldwork night it is clear that considerable numbers of young adults were driving 'under the influence' on Britain's night-time roads, even if at the end of many hours' dancing exertions and after the main effects were declining. These clubbers were not, however, the mobs of drug-crazed drivers one might imagine. Our drivers reported consuming lower amounts of alcohol and drugs than those who were not driving themselves home after the club. For those drivers who did not abstain, there was some expectation that they would have 'sobered up' from their consumption of alcohol and drugs by the end of their night out dancing, combined with an assessment of the state of the individual driver once the club had finished and before setting off. One young woman who was regularly driven home by friends was aware of the road safety issues. 'She does get concerned about the state of mind of the person driving them home after the club. "If they don't look right usually we stay put or we get someone else to drive"'(141113).

For many clubbers, when the club finished the 'sobering up' process began and continued for a considerable length of time, sometimes several hours, either outside the club or at a nearby clubber-friendly cafe or service station where cups of tea, cigarettes, cigarette papers and chewing gum supplies were available. For many, as we have seen in Chapter 4, the ideal come-down or chill-out consumption also included cannabis, alongside the tea and the cigarettes, the depressant or 'downer' to counteract the stimulants or 'uppers'. Clubbers driving home after a night out were fully aware of the need to avoid attracting the attention of night-time police patrols. For those with their own house or flat independent of parents or non-clubbing friends, the sobering-up process could stretch throughout the night and sometimes extend into an impromptu Sunday morning chill-out party (McDermott, 1993). The Leisure Centre staff, for example, reported with some amusement that many clubbers carried on dancing or listening to music played in their car stereos from 2am through until after 5am, when the first Sunday-morning traders arrived in the car park for the car boot sale held in the Leisure Centre at 6am every Sunday morning. Another three hours' dancing might be preferable to immediately driving home, both for the clubbers and for other road users.

These night-time clubbers clustered in cafes and car parks across the region were exposed to added dangers, however. Sitting in a stationary car in the middle of the night has its own risks, including attracting the attention of police patrols and becoming a target of violence, theft or criminal damage from other night owls. One respondent explained how:

> He had been sat in a car outside a club with others when another car pulled up. He and his friends were staring because of drugs they had taken and someone got out of the car and pointed a gun at their car. They quickly drove off. (010705)

Modes of transport home from clubs are directly affected by the location of individual clubs and the various modes of transport which are available and affordable. Taxis proved to be expensive and elusive, public transport was limited, leaving nearly half of clubbers planning to get home by private car. Clubbers discussed the attempts that they made to minimise the risks of such behaviour by nominating abstainers to drive, consuming drugs earlier in the evening, and extending the evening beyond club closing time at a nearby cafe or flat in order to 'chill out' before driving home. Nevertheless, the considerable numbers of clubbers who have consumed legal and/or illicit drugs who drive on Britain's night-time roads is cause for concern.

Conclusion

Clubbers were surprisingly forthcoming in their discussions of their experiences of issues of safety, violence and criminality in clubland. Questions about sources of drugs, illegality and drug distribution suggest a blurring of the distinctions between 'user' and 'dealer' for the majority of recreational drug users in millennial Britain. By far the majority of clubbers reported both supplying and received drugs from friends, either free or for money. Combined with over nine in ten dance drug users obtaining their supplies from someone considered to be a 'friend' or 'known' to them, we can see a quite different picture from the mainstream images of 'dealers'. Clubbers had 'dealers' who were friends and friends who were 'dealers' and cultivated such relationships with drug distributors. Our clubbers, many of whom had years' dance club and dance drug experience, wanted to find and keep the friendly, reliable drug distributors known to them, and to avoid the last minute problems of buying unknown drugs from unknown distributors with all the risks they perceived that to involve. Given the variability of street drugs and the difficulties of reliable supply chains, relationships with drug distributors were fostered rather than avoided. Accessing reliable sources of drugs both inside and outside clubs and 'chilling out' during and after the night out were all part of the 'stay safe' strategies of clubbers. Problems reported by clubbers were as likely to relate to being unable to make contact with elusive 'dealers' before a big night out as they were to aggressive or insistent 'dealers' inside clubs. The retail specialists we interviewed and that clubbers spoke of were not the scary gangsters and the 'dodgy dealers' we hear so much about in relation to late 1990s and millennial clubland. By and large the clubbers in this study did not worry about buying illegal drugs or dealing with drug distribution specialists; they were far more concerned about policing and regulation in and around clubland by police and security/door staff.

The focus of police enforcement of drugs legislation in Britain is now moving from possession to supply with the targeting of resources. Many police chiefs have said they will no longer target possession and people will only be arrested for possession if it comes to police attention in the course of their duties. So both the 1971 Misuse of Drugs Act and the application of the law in practice by the police are based on the distinctions of possession and supply. However, as we have seen, for low-level recreational drug use by clubbers these distinctions do not fit with young people's experiences. For a range of reasons we have outlined, there are real incentives, financial and otherwise, for people to buy their drugs in friendship networks, to buy in bulk and redistribute them, whether or not they plan to make any extra profit from such transactions.

This leads us to agree with the recommendation of the Runciman report which came out of the Police Foundation Inquiry into the 1971 Misuse of Drugs Act which called for a new crime. Located somewhere between possession and supply this would recognise the act of clubbing together to buy drugs where one person may be caught in possession of substantial amounts, more than for personal use, but not for commercial sale for profit (Independent Inquiry, 2000). One drawback, however, would be the definition of profit in such legislation. Whilst profit is not the over-riding priority for these friendship networks, users can and do make profits in cash or in kind from economies of scale.

Clubbers' safety concerns focus on other clubbers, security/door staff and police far more than on the 'dealers' and 'gangsters' who appeared to exercise the minds of police and club management. Police, staff and management concern about 'gangsters' focussed on small groups of young 'wannabes' who had gained notoriety for their involvement in flamboyant displays of power to extort concessions at clubs. The behaviour of the 'wannabes' was conceded by some clubs, and fiercely opposed by others. By comparison, the organised retail specialist drug distributors who operated in these clubs kept a low profile and often worked with the knowledge and condonement of bar staff and door staff.

Experiences of intimidation, hassles and harassment by clubbers tended to take the form of verbal rather than physical aggression, often couched in the nebulous term 'bad attitude'. Where concerns strayed beyond verbal aggression, clubbers discussed their experiences of excessive searches and strip searches by both the police and security/door staff in the hunt for drugs hidden on the person. Clubbers saw this as a clear abuse of power, and the frequency of such reports highlights the need for clarity, regulation and moderation in search policies and procedures both in clubland and on the streets. In general, however, clubbers felt surprisingly safe in and around clubland, and indeed discussed their regular clubbing in terms of a sense of inclusion, safety and feeling 'at home'. For them clubs were 'small bubbles of security in an insecure world' (Bottoms and Wiles, 1995, p. I.20).

The tales of cat and mouse contact with the police on the streets further serve to illustrate the ways in which club space can be seen as safe space for clubbers by comparison with the stop and search tactics of police patrolling conurbations and communities, particularly for our clubbers living on working-class estates and from 'known criminal families'. There is a need for clear regulation and management of clubs in relation to organised criminals, and also to the health, safety and security of hundreds of thousands of clubbers out and about, intoxicated on the streets and in clubland. It appears, however, that the management, policing and regulation of clubland is all too often inconsistent, unpredictable, and symbolic, often in response to pressures from the media, the local authorities or the leisure industry. Strategies for improving this situation include strengthening the Pub and Club Watch for owners and managers, and strengthening and updating customer standards through policies such as the Safer Dancing guidelines for clubbers adopted by Manchester City Council (Newcombe, 1994) and Home Office advice (ACMD, 1994).

Transport is a key issue for the facilitation of clubbers' safety. Taxis were either unavailable or unaffordable for many clubbers and were seen as a problem, with considerable numbers of clubbers having had frustrations and bad experiences with taxis in the past. Public transport proved to be non-existent outside big cities and inconvenient or unreliable within them. This resulted in nearly half of clubbers using private cars to get home from clubs, a finding of particular concern in relation to road traffic safety. The numbers of clubbers driving on Britain's night-time roads who have consumed legal and/or illicit drugs is cause for concern, although their attempts to minimise the risks of such behaviour and the low level of reported accidents is heartening. Clubbers have strong motivation to go clubbing and hundreds of thousands of young people need safe and reasonably priced transport to and from dance venues. The issue to address, therefore, is not a new peel of punitive measures to police Britain's roads but the prospect of affordable alternatives in the form of public transport and organised private-hire taxis, minibuses and coaches.

The clubbers we spoke to negotiated the city streets more or less successfully, made decisions and had strategies to stay safe whilst out clubbing. There were possibilities of incidents with club staff, the police, organised criminals and other clubbers, but clubbers tried to wind their way between all these to have a good night out. And most did. Consequently the club was perceived by them, primarily, not as a location of danger and violence, but as a play space and safe place.

7 The Case for Managing 'Serious' Recreational Drug Use

Complex and contrary

The clubbers who use dance drugs at the weekends are genuinely difficult to characterise and classify. There is so little research knowledge about them and their age peers' drug use, few previous attempts at describing their lifestyles and drugs consumption habits and even less information about their health. They generally have drugs histories or pathways from early adolescence which separate them from the majority of their peers and whilst their drugs antecedents are similar to those of problem drug users, they clearly do not fit this classification. They avoid heroin and crack cocaine and whilst most are daily smokers, regular drinkers and cannabis users, they reserve most Class A stimulant drug use for the weekends. Moreover, despite their comprehensive disregard for the Misuse of Drugs Act they do not, as an overall population, appear more generally delinquent. They are largely well educated, from all social backgrounds but especially professional groups, and the vast majority are in legitimate, gainful employment.

Further difficulty flows from our lack of knowledge about the long-term health implications of these recreational drugs careers. We are unclear about the neuro-toxic effects of alcohol and poly drug use and of ecstasy in particular. This said, there are clearly considerable immediate 'costs' of psycho-active weekends which could be mediated by more concerted harm reduction–secondary prevention initiatives and a greater commitment to clubbers' health and safer dancing.

Currently, however, government has no coherent strategy to *manage* such serious recreational drug use. This lack of coherence comes in part from the institutionalised dishonesty of the drugs discourse, whereby drugs realities and embarrassing truths are not publicly faced. In fairness, however, the complexities of managing clubland and those who dance on drugs pose far more challenge to the coherence of the UK drugs strategy than do 'addicted' heroin and poly drug users who commit crime to pay demanding drugs bills. The drug strategy has accepted managerial responsibility for problem drug users through enforcement, treatment and interventions in the criminal justice and penal systems. There is no such coherence and commitment to deal with the consequences of serious recreational drug use in general and dance drug use in particular. Essentially this chapter explores how such a strategy could be developed. This is no easy task, however, because the clubbers are genuinely contrary: specifically defiant yet not generally delinquent, sophisticated drug users yet still prone to mishap requiring medical assistance, articulate about the need for responsible self-regulation yet content to drive under the influence of alcohol and illicit drugs on the public highway.

Dance drug use, twentysomethings and normalisation

In the first chapter we noted that there are some signs of post-adolescent and young adult recreational drug use rates increasing slightly. We hypothesised that as drugwise adolescents of the 1990s move into young adulthood they may take some of their adolescent drug involvement with them. With increased drugs availability and extensive benign experience and with the traditional settling-down process being deferred or delayed in post-modern times, we suggested that today's younger adults may extend normalisation. It will be several years before we can fully explore this hypothesis using longitudinal and times series prevalence surveys and attitudinal studies of younger adults but a start can be made.

If we regard the clubbers who predominantly grew up across the 1990s as an indicator of this process, perhaps seeing them as the vanguard, then the normalisation thesis receives much support. Indeed there are many cogent arguments that can be made to support this case. On the other hand there are several reasons why such a conclusion may be insecure or certainly premature.

The clubbers as the vanguard?

The clubbers in this study mostly began their drugs careers in early adolescence. Their drugs journeys mirror those of adolescent drug users by order of initiation; from solvents and cannabis via LSD and amphetamines to ecstasy, in many cases even before they could gain legitimate access to the dance club–night club sector. They clearly utilise the cost-benefit assessments found amongst adolescent drug takers (Parker et al., 1998) but seem with age and experience to further accommodate risk and the negative aspects of regular drug use (Shewan et al., 2000; Winstock, 2000). They have extensive drugs experience and by their twenties take drugs regularly and in fairly clearly self-regulated and sophisticated ways. They classically blur the licit (tobacco and alcohol) with the illicit (cannabis, amphetamines, ecstasy and cocaine). Their before, during and after clubbing drugs repertoires make them the ultimate post-modern consumers.

Whilst dance drug users come from all social backgrounds and whilst undoubtedly we can find settings where the customer base will include a criminogenic profile (Hammersley et al., 1999), the clubbers are otherwise largely conforming citizens in terms of being educated, employed and so on. Whilst they are closer to large-scale retail drug distributors than drugwise adolescents, they too utilise informal friendship networks to obtain their drugs. They give and sell, buy and receive dance drugs within normal social relationships. They defy the Misuse of Drugs Act not out of rebelliousness but because they enjoy taking drugs as part of the consumption of leisure. As model psycho-active consumers they illustrate how, if stimulant drugs and cannabis were decriminalised, drug taking could and would for many remain controlled, recreational and functional. We have heard their articulate voices acknowledging there are costs but still celebrating the role of drugs in work hard–play hard lifestyles.

The argument can thus be made that with so many normative and conformist characteristics and broad social representation, the dance drug users are the vanguard. Where they have gone so more of the going out–time out sector will follow. The reasons for this are many. Firstly, the going out sector is endlessly reinforced by new entrants, from the age of 17, many of whom who are also drugwise. Secondly, those who 'go out' share many of the characteristics of the clubbers being disproportionately smokers and drinkers with drug-trying antecedents. Thirdly, illicit drugs continue to be cheaper and more available. Finally the emergent UK café bar society, with extended licensing hours, late night dancing/music licences, in mimicking and competing with the dance club–night club environment, is providing new arenas for the extension and migration of dance drug use, along with summer holiday resorts and music festivals increasingly dedicated to dance music.

Enigmatic excess?

All this said, and because we remain short of robust supportive data, an alternative case can be made. Normalisation requires cultural accommodation. We see this clearly emerging in respect of cannabis use (Independent Inquiry, 2000) and more equivocally the trying and occasional use of certain stimulant drugs in the general young adult population. But many dance drug users operate well beyond cultural levels of tolerance/toleration. They are enormously drug experienced. They spend large amounts of money on drugs repertoires. They take risks and suffer negative effects in ways which the more cautious majority of their age peers find alarming. They endure the very experiences which abstainers and cautious drug users list as reasons why they will never take amphetamines, ecstasy or cocaine (Parker et al., 1998; Measham et al., 1998b; Boys et al., 2000). Whilst the dance drug users remain discreetly hidden and condoned in clubland and whilst they overtly celebrate their intoxication with fellow users and clubbing drinkers, the chances of their disinhibited 'drug bonding' behaviour being accommodated in other social settings and venues seem remote. If they are a vanguard they are a long way ahead of the main party. More likely they are and will remain a small minority embracing, as discussed in Chapter 1, around 10 per cent of the post-adolescent–young adult population. Their hedonistic excesses, whilst not demanding subcultural explanations, still make them something of an enigma.

A question for the new decade

With such a finely balanced debate its resolution will be slow, mainly because this age group is so scattered and difficult to research, but also because such research is a low priority amongst funders anyway. If the increases in recent drug use amongst young adults continue, say for cocaine (e.g. Corkery, 2000: Ramsay and Partridge, 1999), then we may see some sustained commitment to researching this age group develop amongst commissioners. The immediate prospects for careful monitoring are slight, however, with official priorities elsewhere and within the 'drugs strategy' agenda focussed on crime reduction. This all makes hypotheses testing and forecasting more difficult.

Our own view is that such increases in drug use are likely to occur within the mainstream, young adult, going-out population via a growing variety of social events, parties and café bar society. The committed clubbers and dance drug users, whilst they may well take advantage of this diffusion, will, we think, still by choice, remain loyal customers of the 'real' clubs. Their profiles and behaviour meet the normalisation criteria – drugs availability, drug use rates, sophisticated and comfortable with drug use, blurring the licit and illicit – until we demand the accommodation of their behaviour by less drug involved and abstentious peers. We have very little evidence either way on this dimension but what there is, for example the tolerance shown by 'drug free' clubbers, is not sufficient to make the case for widespread moral/social accommodation. For this reason alone we remain ambivalent about recruiting the clubbers' drugs profile to support notions of the extension of the normalisation of recreational drug use. They will only be significant actors in normalisation if their more cautious, non-clubbing peers begin to embrace or tolerate aspects of a 'time out' style which combine alcohol and drugs in a similar way. Currently we simply do not know what the attitudes and views of the general young adult population are beyond occasional public attitude surveys.

The enforcement agenda

During the 1990s amidst the 'moral panic' about ecstasy use and unofficial 'raves' and festivals, we saw the classic law and order response to dance clubs and dance drug use. Numerous legislative and licensing measures were implemented in this period, such as the 1994 Criminal Justice and Public Order Act which amongst other things included a wide range of measures which effectively criminalised open-air dance parties and unlicensed events and the young people even travelling to them (Measham et al., 1998a). More recently these measures have been extended to allow local authorities and the police to refuse licenses and thus close down clubs and venues which are regarded as having a 'serious drugs problem', either on the premises or nearby land (1997 Public Entertainment Licences (Drug Misuse) Act). From time to time local, political or media pressure to clamp down on errant clubland emerges and the local police undertake fairly intensive operations. They search queues, walk through clubs armed and in flak jackets and/or mount undercover operations inside clubs. We witnessed no fewer than three different unco-ordinated police operations in one of the fieldwork clubs on the same weekend. This inspectorial and 'final warning' approach to managing clubland is required, particularly if clubs are managed or financed or excessively influenced by organised criminals or those whose standards of safety and security are inadequate. The problem however, as we discussed in the last chapter, is that all this is *ad hoc* and inconsistent. It is often symbolic: an enforcement gesture because in reality the clubs cannot be comprehensively policed by the local force. There are far more pressing demands, particularly at weekends. In the end the clubs are expected to self-regulate and employ their own security and door staff. Indeed club staff regularly complain that the police won't even turn up when requested to deal with a drugs incident or with intimidation of club staff by 'organised criminals'.

The truth, spoken only in private, is that the police have neither the resources nor the inclination to enforce the Misuse of Drugs Act. They incidentally produce more than enough drugs possessions through routine policing and stop and search and so usually limit their proactive intervention to major or politically sensitive incidents and requests for intervention from other key players in the local government apparatus.

All this corresponds with the clubbers' reportage. One in five have drugs cautions or convictions, mainly possession, accumulated over the years of being out and about. Whilst over their pubbing–clubbing careers half our clubbers have at some time or other felt threatened or harassed – be it by other clubbers, club staff, dealers or the police – overall they claim to feel pretty safe and secure on their weekends out. There is no sense that they regard going to town and clubbing as a dangerous past-time. This dominant reality is lost in public discourse which focusses on and collates the mishaps and disorder. The fact that hundreds of thousands of young people go out clubbing every weekend, have a 'brilliant' time and get home safely week in, week out is hardly headline news. Yet were this not the case the enduring popularity of such leisure-time adventures and the growth of town and city centre night-time visitors would not occur and 24-hour cities would have no prospect of becoming a reality.

Turning to the national drugs strategy we find little clarification or guidance as to whether this local approach is strategically sound. Whilst the national strategy encourages local decision making to resolve local problems, we might expect some guidance to ensure consistency, natural justice and best enforcement practice – given current inconsistencies in the way drugs are policed. This, however, is noticeable by its absence. Clearly the aspirational goals of reducing the availability and use of Class A drugs will embrace the clubbers and imply targeted policing of both supply and – presumably – possession. But again no thought or guidance is given to how this should be achieved and what might be the consequences, both intentional and unintentional. The one clear sign of managerial engagement is in respect of driving under the influence of drugs and the strategy specifically prioritises regulatory developments in this arena.

In conclusion, the enforcement agenda for clubland is interpreted at the local level and its style and intensity will depend not just on policing resources and priorities but the influence of other key groups including drugs agencies, the local media, local political parties and local authority partnerships. The problem with all this is that delegation produces inconsistencies and injustices and from time to time clampdowns on clubland which, whilst they may make gains from a licensing or policing perspective, can have serious unintended consequences. The dance clubs and night clubs contain, even segregate, the serious dance drug users from the wider going out population. Closing them will either transfer 'the problem' to another area with more clubs or, if they are in short supply, displace and disperse the dance drug users into café bar society and the wider party scene. This may, ironically, encourage the very extension of Class A drug use which the 'purge' was presumably meant to discourage as drug users and drinkers mingle whilst the music plays on.

We do not suggest that there are easy answers to this conundrum; on the contrary this is the point. It is simply not possible in a resource-finite, democratic society with such high rates of recreational drug use to enforce the law effectively. It is as well that despite the 'bad' things that do happen around clubs and drugs (Morris, 1998), these arenas and their customers generally cause little trouble. Moreover, what trouble there is relates more to alcohol than illicit drugs (Wise, 1997), as recent crime figures suggest.

Towards the management of serious recreational drug use

The public health imperative

The absence of an overall strategy to manage the negative impact of serious recreational drug use may seem unfathomable to some. How can a society with one of the highest rates of drug use and the most extensive dance club–dance drug scenes in the world not have developed a national strategy or, more strangely, *have* a national drugs strategy but remain effacive and evasive about such a key issue? The answer is found at the heart of politics, whereby the 'war on drugs' discourse and the forces of conservatism in both previous Conservative and current New Labour administrations have undermined and censored public debate. There is institutionalised dishonesty throughout government in respect of the drugs issue. Private and public discourses are poles apart and the more open-minded and rational private perspectives – of politicians, civil servants, enforcers, local officials – are rarely publicly aired. Indeed doing so is likely to damage the whistleblower's career. This is essentially why the drugs strategy refuses to fully discuss the management of recreational drug use. To admit that much Class A drug use is not linked to criminal careers, that large numbers of 'respectable' people manage their dance drug use successfully and that there is no prospect of effectively enforcing the drugs laws in the pubbing/clubbing sector, is to admit defeat in the 'war on drugs' and to be accused by the tabloid media of going soft on hard drugs. To officially and openly sanction harm minimisation and public health measures for clubbers is to agree that such drug use is widespread and that with some 'really useful' guidance and regulation probably no more immediately risky than many outdoor pursuits. The public health imperative is thus uniquely muffled in respect of recreational drug use. It is acceptable for problem drug users who can be medicalised or seen as a wider health threat to the public but for 'normal' people, with no excuses, then the response must primarily be enforcement. Carefully considered calls to review the Misuse of Drugs Act in respect of reclassifying ecstasy and rethinking legal definitions of drug dealing – 'sorting' friends – are thus dismissed (Independent Inquiry, 2000).

This is why the management of recreational drug use has not developed from the centre. It is also why government, whilst maintaining the public 'no discussion, no compromise' position, also quietly sanctions local harm minimisation initiatives and 'safer dancing' programmes (Branigan and Wellings, 1999). Because of a lack of national guidance and encouragement, however, such initiatives are currently patchy and inadequate. This impasse thus relates more to the State than the dance drug users. There are the embryonic signs that government may engage with the realities of clubland but this will be, as we discuss later, initially focussed on drug driving. A post-election tiptoe into harm minimisation may follow but with the usual linguistic gymnastics to camouflage this progress, notably defining the clubbers as a 'vulnerable group' alongside care leavers and homeless people! In the next section we outline a more substantive harm minimisation–health promotion agenda based on what the clubbers who participated in this study have highlighted and revealed.

Harm minimisation and health promotion

One of the most frustrating realities for those protecting and promoting public health is the collective refusal or difficulty for a significant minority of the population to do as they have been told. Healthy diets, regular exercise, no smoking, moderate drinking, no illicit drug use, safer sex are all messages regularly sent to the public, especially through lifestyle magazines, television programmes, news reports and government campaigns.

The clubbers are, as ever, contrary. Thanks to their dance floor exertions they are fairly fit (Crank et al., 1999) yet we have seen that the body mass assessments make them disproportionately slim citizens, which at the extremes may be a health issue (Winstock, 2000). Yet nearly seven in ten smoke, almost all are regular drinkers and they routinely smoke cannabis and consume moderate quantities of stimulant drugs at weekends. Moreover much of this is done in combination, thereby increasing neurotoxicity (Shewan et al., 2000; POST, 1996).

Given their educational backgrounds and socio-economic profiles, it is reasonable to assume that the majority of the country's clubbers are quite able to take responsibility for their personal health. Indeed their elaborate strategies to rest and recover, to cut down on psycho-active consumption, seek medical advice, and so on, support this. In short, this is a population which is potentially likely to be susceptible to public health information.

Unfortunately, communicating with the clubbers in a way they might recognise and accept is challenging and, for government, potentially politically damaging and in truth at odds with the operational thrust of the national drugs strategy. This said, the starting-point for a strategy would have to be that their essential mix of alcohol and dance drugs is non-negotiable because the benefits of psycho-active weekends are rated too highly. The regularity of attendance, the expenditure and the time commitment made by our respondents bear witness to the significance of this illegal leisure. Thus any information, advice, discussion and guidance must orbit around this nexus.

Helpfully, as well as promoting the health of clubbers, any national programme would be able to argue that a secondary gain would be reducing costs to the National Health Service, particularly in respect of Accident and Emergency pressures and costs but also in respect of 'unproductive' consultancy in primary health settings, given patients' economy with the truth.

There are numerous ways to develop such a strategy and when we bring together the scattered *ad hoc* research and good practice in respect of safer clubbing as did the Club Health 2000 conference in Amsterdam, we realise that it is only a lack of political will to co-ordinate and resource such a programme which is missing. In suggesting a three-legged approach we simply offer one way of assembling key information. There are many other structures available (e.g. Scottish Drugs Forum, 1998).

The *night out* agenda is the most difficult to specify because the most cautious and thus 'safest' advice – don't drink too much alcohol, don't mix alcohol with drugs, don't mix drugs, don't keep redosing or topping up – conflicts with the essential elements of the night out. More realistically the harm minimisation message needs to be about finding one's limits and what are the right combinations of alcohol and drugs for each individual. We noted that periods of abstinence after over-indulging on amphetamines was high on the self-regulatory priorities of our clubbers which is in line with clinical observations (Williamson et al., 1997) and sustained research with stimulant users (Klee and Morris, 1994). A range of examples of repertoires or styles of consumption which tend to lead to bad outcomes is thus needed. Some of these will be recognised and person-alised, thereby gaining credibility. For example, coke-heads who drink strong lager become hyper, sometimes aggressive. If the E's too strong you need to sit down, chill out, even go home or you'll make a fool of yourself, perhaps putting yourself in vulnerable situations or risky encounters or ruin everyone else's night out as well. Have a plan and a limit before you go out and endorse it with sensible friends. If you're depressed don't expect automatic relief. Remember intoxicated decisions are often bad decisions. Smart clubbers don't screw up so don't 'neck' anything available via strangers. Don't take Viagra if you've been sniffing poppers is another important piece of advice given the contra-indicators of nitrites and Sildenafil. Have plans to get home which don't involve drink/drug driving. Never leave friends unaccounted for. Know your first aid in case someone has a fit or gets 'monged'.

The *recovery and review* agenda is currently underdeveloped both in terms of educating clubbers about personal health matters but also social health issues. Remembering the range for recovery from a clubbing weekend is one to seven days but with an average of 1.7 days, the recovery problems declared by four in ten clubbers were important. They revolved around 'performance' the following week in terms of tiredness, concentration or memory loss, mood swings leading to absence or lateness for work/study, and personal or professional relationships being adversely affected (Shewan et al., 2000). For a small minority serious psychological difficulties were disclosed.

Many recreational drug users modify their drugs consumption when they have to face forthcoming events such as academic exams, job interviews or key deadlines at work. The recovery agenda would again tune in to this self-regulation or lack of it, reminding the audience that they or those close to them might be negatively affected. Clubbing hair stylists sometimes advise that Mondays and Saturdays are when they cut their worst styles but more significantly what of those who work in key services who are public transport drivers, doctors, nurses, engineers, mechanics and so on? The agenda should attempt to appeal to their social responsibilities and encourage them to use flexi-time, Friday nights to go clubbing, though in practice the 'sicky' day off may well become more popular than it already is.

Practical information about milky drinks and fruit juice, isotonic sports drinks (without vodka) as replacement fluids, eating healthily, resetting the body clock and keeping supple would all find their way into this agenda, along with listing the likely unwanted effects of a heavy weekend.

The recovery period is when clubbers should review the impact of dancing on drugs in respect of physical and particularly psychological well being. It is perhaps on the Wednesday after a heavy weekend that if morbidity is setting in they may best recognise this, given that the immediate consequential effects should be disappearing and more endemic problems thus become identifiable. Their current problem, like that of those around them and indeed generalist health agency staff, is that the negative signs and symptoms of regular or high-dose 'recreational' drug use are not well known. A whole range of minor 'problems' may be drug-related and would disappear with moderation or abstention but the symptoms – blurred vision, headaches, digestive tract problems, insomnia, lethargy and so on – are difficult to relate to drug use if the 'facts' are little known. This brings us to the development of an ongoing health agenda.

The *broader health* agenda is the most difficult to implement because it requires some retraining of primary health care workers, particularly GPs and helpline staff. The key thrust of this component involves providing awareness of the dangers and side-effects of stimulant drug use and identifying them 'early'. There are quite clearly certain medical conditions and predispositions (Verheyden and Curran, 1999) which make dancing on drugs dangerous and this should be highlighted, for instance, to asthmatics, diabetics, epileptics and people with cardio-vascular problems. We also have concerns about the scale and intensity of mental health problems reported by a substantial minority of the interview sample. We cannot describe from this study the exact nature of co-morbidity but the case studies discussed in Chapter 5 are salutary and suggest that psychological distress and mental health problems are prevalent amongst some clubbers.

All this information needs consistently updating to deal with new drugs, newly popular drugs and combinations, and new information about the longer-term effects of stimulant drugs and poly drug use. Currently this information – advice, aside from scattered local clubbers' initiatives, is generated by drugwise clubbers and recreational drug users themselves through endlessly swapping drugs stories. But the information is potentially inaccurate or incomplete and anyway takes time to build up, especially for new entrants to the scene. So for instance the rapidly increasing popularity of cocaine at the start of the new decade (Corkery, 2000) will eventually generate drugs wisdom about the scale and nature of the casualty list. Drugs stories and discussions will focus on bingeing, hyper behaviour, domestic grief, psychological distress, bleeding noses and celebrity disfigurement as a small casualty rate emerges. Using heroin as a chill out drug must primarily be challenged, the reasons given and alternative depressants recommended (Handy et al., 1998). It is essential to inform this drug wisdom more accurately, more fully and more rapidly.

The difficulty with all this is whether primary health care and the main helplines are capable of dealing with such 'presentations': 23 per cent of our interview sample had consulted a doctor about symptoms they believed to be related to alcohol or illicit drugs. Many appear not to have disclosed their drugs status (see also Parker et al., 1998) thereby possibly undermining the diagnosis and treatment regime. Poor appetite, insomnia, feeling hyper, spotty complexion and mood swings are unlikely to trigger the average family doctor into diagnosing cocaine 'misuse'. Whilst Accident and Emergency staff have, through increasing clinical experience, come to recognise the costs of alcohol and drug misadventures (Luke et al., 1999), it is unrealistic to expect most family doctors to spot underlying morbidity, especially if they are not told the full facts. However this is the crux of the problem; the doctor may know the 'family' and have treated the clubbers since they were children. The need to reaffirm the integrity of patient–doctor relationships and the importance of confidentiality for all staff throughout the local medical centre is a prerequisite to honest consultation. The alternative – easily accessible drugs advice and treatment services with expert knowledge of dance drugs – simply do not exist in sufficient numbers to create uniform service delivery. This is a further reason to communicate directly with and educate clubbers.

In conclusion, it is quite possible to develop an additional component to the national drugs strategy which focusses on recreational drug use. The forces of conservatism have undermined this however, and so once again official responses lag behind drugs realities. The role of government should be to sanction, encourage and finance such an initiative and provide guidelines for implementation. It would not be difficult to create demonstration projects built on local good practice in collaborative arrangements for safer dancing, producing leaflets and flyers for clubbers (e.g. Scottish Drugs Forum; Crew 2000; HIT, Lifeline) and encouraging clubs to be proactive in respect of working with other agencies. The only missing ingredient is official pragmatic realism.

Regulation and public safety

As a direct consequence of the primacy of the enforcement agenda which was the foundation of the first attempt at a drugs strategy in the mid-1990s, we find government has already accepted some responsibility for the management of recreational drug use. There can be no quarrel with this as the evidence builds about drug use and driving (AA, 1998), and drug use and the after-effects at work (Health and Safety Executive, 1998). This study, given its scale, offers important corroboration about driving home from clubland and going to work or study during the recovery period. There are major practical and then legal issues ahead in rolling out such regulatory measures, however. Effective roadside drug tests are several years away and the proof that illicit drug use causes an impairment which in turn contributes to, for instance, an accident, will be difficult to deliver to the courts. This is why we suggested that social responsibility should be emphasised in our earlier public health proposals.

Most importantly of all however, the overall management strategy needs broadening. Currently there are inadequate organisational arrangements for offering the time out population adequate and appropriate alternative transport options, whether public or contracted to private companies. There should be a concerted effort to create a transport system which can take night owls home safely. Depending on circumstances, the ingredients would include creating more night buses, contracting Hackney and private-hire taxi companies to provide regular services and encouraging clubs and café bars to create a minibus system. Subsidising clubber networks, for example, with entry ticket reduction vouchers to hire local minibuses and coaches to take them to the popular long distance venues, whereby the drivers stay at the venue and ensure all the passengers return to the transport and get home safely, could be particularly effective. We already see these kinds of initiatives for certain festivals such as 'Creamfields' in Liverpool and larger hardcore dance events, but this approach of taking responsibility for clubbers' safety should be routine, every weekend, practice.

The notion of drug testing in the workplace is already explored in the national drugs strategy. There can be little doubt that however controversial all this will be, we will see a gradual extension of testing. The dilemma for the dance drug users, over and above testing positive for cannabis with its long half life, is that they may produce a positive test for amphetamines, MDMA or cocaine. They could argue that their psycho-active weekends were separate from their employment arrangements but on their own self-reports a sizeable minority would be being economical with the truth.

Risk, health and hedonism

The desire for hedonism at weekends has a long and robust tradition, with the dance club just the most recent manifestation of this broader night-club tradition. As the leisure landscape continues to evolve there will undoubtedly be new styles of consumption and related venues. Most immediately the further deregulation of licensing hours and the development of very late licence café bars means the dance clubs and night clubs' monopoly on post-midnight psycho-active leisure is already broken. This, we have argued, may well see the dispersal and diffusion of dance drug use into more mainstream young adult licensed leisure venues. The extension of cocaine use is the most likely immediate outcome given the compatibility of cocaine and alcohol for many users. This said, the 'night club' will adapt and survive because it will allow consecutive age cohorts of devotees to drink and take their dance drugs with relative impunity and for them in an exciting, yet comfortable, accepting social environment.

The risks that clubbers take may appear daunting, even foolhardy, to more cautious, older heads. The conventional view is that those with jobs, degrees and respectable families should know better than to risk their reputations and health dancing on drugs. This is why enforcement is such an attractive feature in the drugs debate. It is the most direct way of dealing with defiance and deviance. However, if enforcement cannot be adequately administered, which is the case with recreational drug use, and if apparent outright disobedience is merely a by-product of popular cultural consumption, then a different per-spective is required to manage this drug-using sector.

We have implicitly situated our exploration of the motives and behaviour of clubbers on a 'risk society' backcloth. Our informants live in rapidly changing, uncertain economic and social milieux. They embrace the pace and try to stay with it. They speed up and slow down with the chemical aids so readily available in their social space. Their dance drugs make weekend nights last longer, their depressants persuade body clocks to ignore Sunday-light. These play-hard weekends are in relative harmony with studying or working and living ordinary weekday lives. Why work all week if you can't look forward to brilliant weekends?

It is of course neither this simple nor this efficient. Prices are paid and there is a casualty rate, particularly amongst the youngest clubbers (17–20 years) who quickly take up fully-blown dance drug repertoires yet lack sophisticated drugs wisdom about harm minimisation and coping strategies, thereby suffering the most harms. However, unless we can grasp the integrity of the motives and experiences of the dance drug users and their commitment to their post-modern lifestyles, we have little prospect of developing an effective, equitable strategy which balances rights with responsibilities and control with appropriate care.

A coherent management strategy

In conclusion, illegal drug use in the going out sector is now so widespread and the profile of the clubbers so representative of all socio-economic backgrounds that all this represents a major challenge to the State. Government, through institutionalised dishonesty, has got itself into an untenable position. It has an enforcement agenda which is practically impossible to implement and yet refuses to accept its fundamental role in managing the negative consequences of widespread recreational drug use – the public health and 'health and safety' agendas. It will readily take on responsibilities which fit the drugs enforcement agenda such as inspecting premises, vetting door staff, closing down clubs and pubs, but it is quite unable to extend this to produce a comprehensive management approach. We have no quarrel with developing drink/drug driving and drugs at work enforcement as these protect both the clubbers and of course the general public from socially irresponsible drug use. Badly-run clubs or clubs with strong connections with organised crime need to be comprehensively 'policed'. The missing elements of a coherent management strategy involve providing the clubbers, as tax-paying, generally law-abiding citizens, with infor-mation, advice and assistance to minimise the harm that may accrue from their drugs decisions and to at least ensure they make reasonably informed choices. We do not deny other 'offenders' such a service nor do we refuse to attribute full citizenship to those who 'misuse' tobacco or alcohol or indeed food.

Recent social history reminds us that where we have a dissonance between the law and normative citizen behaviour then 'the problem' endlessly resurfaces in media and public discourses until it is resolved or an acceptable compromise reached. We have seen alcohol's immense popularity produce such cultural antithesis and defeat prohibition. With ongoing secularisation has come the deregulation of licensing hours, beginning with Sunday opening, then all-day and now late-night opening. We saw consumer and commercial pressure finally undermine restricted trading times whereby seven-day shopping has become a reality. The age of consent for homosexual relationships has been lowered as gay rights have gradually gained strength. Yet all these 'deviant' hedonistic behaviours were wholly condemned 35 years ago and enforcement was often quite punitive for transgressors.

The drugs issue is coming under similar pressure, primarily in respect of the decriminalisation of cannabis, the reclassifying of ecstasy and revised definitions of drugs possession and supply (Independent Inquiry, 2000). The opposition is primarily ideological and political once again. The dysfunctions in governance that flow from a refusal to engage in rational debate and identify *specific* changes in the drugs laws and enforcement agenda and to facilitate public health and citizen welfare are becoming increasingly transparent as recreational drug use expands and its accommodation slowly grows.

The creation of a balanced, coherent approach to managing serious recreational drug use in the going out sector is tenable with political will and sophistication. There are numerous local examples which have developed *de facto* without a central steer, where local authorities, the police, harm minimisation-oriented drugs agencies and club owners have developed safer clubbing – for instance in Greater London and Liverpool. Even without revised legislation a national programme could develop with a change of political heart within government. Once again we are left identifying the forces of conservatism at the centre as being indirectly responsible for undermining the public health and safety imperative in favour of political goals locked on to the 'war on drugs' and the politics of re-election.

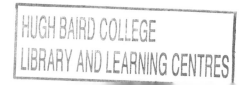

Notes

1 Excessive Appetites? Young Britons and Recreational Drug Use

1. Orford, J. (1985) *Excessive Appetites: A psychological view of addictions*, Wiley: Chichester.

2 Identity and Location in Clubland: Gender, Class, Race, Sexual Orientation and Club Culture

1. An amended version of this chapter appears in Measham (2000).
2. The history of the policing of dance clubs is exemplified in the opening, closing and policing of the legendary Hacienda, a dance club in Manchester city centre which has entered twentieth-century folklore as the original acid house venue and the dance centre of Europe, at its height attracting dance tourists from around the globe. The two-pronged assault on dance clubs by the police and local authorities, of clamping down on illegal 'raves' and allowing licensed venues to stay open longer, then clamping down on licensed clubs and allowing bars to stay open longer, will be discussed in more detail in Chapters 6 and 7. For a detailed history of the inception and demise of the Hacienda and the 'Madchester' scene, see, for example, Reynolds (1998), Garratt (1998), Collin and Godfrey (1997) and Redhead (1993).
3. From Dionysus or Bacchus (also known as the Lord of Dance, the God of Ecstasy), the ancient Greek god of ecstatic liberation, sensuality, wine and intoxication. His followers participated in ritualised activities involving music, dance, orgiastic sex and intoxicants to achieve altered states of consciousness.
4. Redhead, 1993, p. 4.
5. For a discussion of the division of labour in drugs supply whereby the gender, race and class divisions of wider society are reproduced in the drugs economy see Maher (1997). Her ethnography of black female drug users and sex workers in New York concludes that the illegal drugs economy is a gender-stratified labour market which operates with constraints, norms and cultures as does any workplace.

> Institutionalized sexism in the underworld was the most powerful element shaping women's experiences in the drug economy: it inhibited their access to drug-business work roles and effectively foreclosed their participation as higher-level distributors. ... The formal organizational characteristics of highly-structured drug markets, the distribution networks which sustain them, and the cultural practices and beliefs of the social actors who inhabit them, work together to foster both sex/gender and race/ethnic segmentation in the (illegal) workplace. (Maher, 1997, pp. 106–7)

6. See McDermott for verbatim quotes from a Liverpool builder whose first ecstasy tablet at a stag night led to him dancing for hours with fellow builders. He did not drink alcohol, then returned home at 3am to face his partner's jealousy and disbelief that he had only been dancing with male friends, with all of them sober, dancing together for hours (1993, p. 218).

7. See Saunders (1997) for a discussion of the medical and sociological research on the effects of ecstasy on sexual desire and sexual behaviour. He concludes that: ' ... a universal effect of the drug is to remove male sexual aggression ... People on ecstasy become more sensual and less lustful' (Saunders, 1997, p. 57).

8. For quotes from young women illustrating this see Henderson, 1993b, p. 50. For example, one young woman said 'We just spent ages together like kissing and being teenagerish. ... It was great because I was at a rave and there was no chance of having sex or anything and it was quite a secure sort of feeling. I just sat in a corner and snogged for quite a long time. Being cuddled and massaged and stuff and it was lovely' (19-year-old female respondent, quoted in Henderson, 1993b, p. 50).

9. Ecstasy or MDMA is sometimes allocated to the family of drugs called 'empathogens'. In 1983 Metzner proposed this new name for a group of substances called phenethylamines, including MDMA, MMDA, MDEA and MDA, whose effects were empathy-inducing rather than psychedelic (Eisner, 1989; Shulgin and Shulgin, 1991).

10. In the house and garage scene, behaviour linked with excessive stimulant consumption became passé (Measham et al., 1998). When Danny and Jenni Rampling held the last Shoom in November 1989 Danny Rampling explained their reasoning for its closure: 'Everything began to get a bit sordid, seedy and frightening. People had started to let themselves go ... Unfortunately people were starting to lose it a bit.' So the Ramplings opened a new club night called Pure, with a more dressy door policy and discouragement of the excesses of Shoom: 'It wasn't a real authoritarian policy ... It was more just, *let's smarten things up a bit*. The whole nation had become baggy. Everyone was conforming to this look that had been a non-conformist thing in the beginning' (Danny Rampling, quoted in Garratt, 1998, p. 242).

11. The fundamental role of passion in causing madness is illustrated by François Boissier de Sauvages, quoted in Foucault (1961, p. 85): 'The distraction of our mind is the result of our blind surrender to our desires, our incapacity to control or to moderate our passions ... these excesses in eating, in drinking, these indispositions, these corporeal vices which cause madness, the worst of all maladies' (1772, p. 12).

12. Although Reynolds sees the defining feature of jungle as class rather than race:

> The true meaning of 'junglist' is defined not by race, but by class, in so far as all working-class urban youth are 'niggas' in the eyes of authority. Junglist youth constitute a kind of internal colony within the United Kingdom: a ghetto of labour surplus to the economy's requirements, of potential criminals under surveillance and guilty-until-proven-innocent as far as the Law is concerned. (Reynolds, 1997, pp. 248–9)

13. The most famous attack on a gay bar was the police raid and subsequent 'Stonewall riots' at Stonewall Inn, Christopher Street, Greenwich Village, New York in June 1969 (Weeks, 1979). One of the most recent attacks on a gay bar was the bombing of the Admiral Duncan pub at Old Compton Street, Soho, London, in April 1999 by an anti-gay extremist individual.

4 The Clubbers and their Nights Out

1. Socio-economic class was coded using the ESRC/ONS new Review of Government Social Classifications (1998). The new SEC classification is '(1) based on a widely-accepted conceptual model which has been established as robust by researchers in diverse fields and in many countries; (2) hierarchical, so that a full version of the classification may be collapsed in several ways into analytic variables for use in policy

and academic research; (3) flexible in terms of the quality of data required for its implementation; (4) clear in terms of rules for including the non-employed population; and (5) maintained through explicit procedures' (p. xi).

2. A 'past 3 month' prevalence question was used in the sweep survey (N=2,057) rather than the more usual 'past month' question (the latter was employed in the in-depth interviews). Although this reduces comparability with other surveys, it was essential in the sweep survey because the past three month criterion was used to define regular dance drug use for our purposes (see Chapter 2), serving to 'filter respondents, rather than used simply to produce descriptive statistics'.

3. A unit of alcohol is the UK standard unit of 10 ml (8 grammes) alcohol. One unit is equal to approximately one half pint of 4% ABV beer/lager; or, one 24 ml measure of 40% ABV spirit; or, one 125 ml glass of 12% ABV table wine.

4. The coding of typical amounts consumed was straightforward for ecstasy, and coded simply as number of tablets consumed. However, it should be noted that strength of tablets are likely to have varied, typically from 60mg to 140mg. Users mostly reported amounts of amphetamine consumed in grammes, although again, strength and purity will have varied. Where users reported consumption of amphetamines in 'dabs', we estimated that there were approximately 20 dabs per gramme. Where users reported consumption of cocaine in 'lines', we estimated that there were approximately 20 lines to a gramme of cocaine.

5 From Coping Strategies to Health Costs

1. Length of stay in the club was calculated by subtracting the time of the initial sweep interview, conducted usually as club goers entered the club, or shortly thereafter, for the majority of respondents, from the time of the club closing. Length of stay ranged from 0.33 hours to 7 hours with a mean of 3.8 hours (sd = 1.15). This represents an average length of stay: although some club goers will have left the club prior to its closing, for others, the sweep interview was conducted later than on entry into the club.

2. Policing and illegality concerns included: official responses to drug use and concerns around the purchase of drugs. Psychological problems included: depression and related responses; amnesia/vagueness; panic attacks/anxiety; paranoia; fears about surroundings; unpleasant hallucinations and artificiality of emotions. Social problems included: concerns for others; sexual risk taking; concerns about dancing; concerns about violence; concerns about habitual drug taking; concerns about socialising and boredom. Physical problems included: blurred vision/dizziness; fatigue/lack of energy; insomnia/sleeping problems; stomach pain/digestive disorders; vomiting; weight/appetite problems; mouth-related problems and dehydration.

3. Examination of bivariate relationships here and elsewhere involved conducting several hundred tests of statistical significance. Using tests of statistical significance as a guide to exploring relationships amongst variables can be misleading because, using the $p < 0.05$ level of significance, we should expect that 1 in 20 relationships will be significant by chance alone. There are two reasons why this approach is nevertheless employed here: firstly, the research is exploratory given that there is little available research to use for theory-driven hypothesis testing. Secondly, in spite of the number of bivariate relationships tested, only those relationships for which we have reasonable grounds, by way of insights gained from fieldwork, available evidence from other sources, as well as hunches and intuitions, are examined.

4. As discussed in Chapter 3, we had reason to believe that a considerable proportion of club goers who reported their sexual orientation as 'bisexual', particularly at the

City Centre club, were actually heterosexual. Although data are presented for each of the three categories, only differences between gay/lesbian and straight respondents will be discussed.

5. Analysis of the medical assessments was carried out by Dr Duncan Raistrick, Clinical Director, Leeds Addiction Unit.

Bibliography

Advisory Council on the Misuse of Drugs (1994) *Drug Misusers and the Criminal Justice System, Part II: Police, Drug Misusers and the Community*, London: HMSO.

Akram, G. (1997) *Patterns of Use and Safety Awareness amongst Users of Dance Drugs in Nottingham*, Master of Public Health, Nottingham: University of Nottingham.

Akram, G. and Galt, M. (1999) 'A profile of harm-reduction practices and co-use of illicit and licit drugs amongst users of dance drugs' *Drugs: Education, Prevention and Policy* 6(2):215–25.

Alciati, A., Scaramelli, B., Fusi, A., Butteri, E., Cattaneo, M.L. and Mellado, C. (1999) 'Three cases of delirium after "ecstasy" ingestion' *Journal of Psychoactive Drugs* 31(2):167–70.

Aldridge, J. and Measham, F. (1999) 'Sildenafil (Viagra) is used as a recreational drug in England' *British Medical Journal*, 318:669 (6 March).

Aldridge, J., Parker, H. and Measham, F. (1998) *Patterns and Profiles of Young People's 'Recreational' Drug Use and the Feasibility of Identifying Risk Factors*, Report to the Drugs Prevention Initiative, London: Home Office.

Aldridge, J., Parker, H. and Measham, F. (1999) *Drug Trying and Drug Use Across Adolescence*, DPAS Paper 1, London: Home Office.

Anthony, W. (1998) *Class of 88: The True Acid House Experience*, London: Virgin.

Ashton, C. and Kamali, F. (1995) 'Personality, lifestyles, alcohol and drug consumption in a sample of British medical students' *Medical Education* 29:187–92.

Automobile Association (1998) *Drugs and Driving; a Discussion Paper*, Group Public Policy, Basingstoke: Automobile Association.

Balding, J. (1999) *Young People in 1998*, Exeter: Exeter University.

Banerjea, K. and Barn, J. (1996) 'Versioning terror: Jallianwala Bagh and the jungle', in Sharma, S., Hutnyk, J. and Sharma, A. (eds), *Dis-orienting Rhythms: The Politics of the New Asian Dance Music*, London: Zed.

Barnard, M., Forsyth, A. and McKeganey, N. (1996) 'Levels of drug use among a sample of Scottish schoolchildren' *Drugs: Education, Prevention and Policy* 3(1):81–96.

Benson, R. (1996) 'Moving House', *The Face*, July, reproduced in Benson, R. (ed.), (1997) *Night Fever: Club Writing in* The Face *1980–1997*, London: Boxtree.

Benson, R. (ed.), (1997) *Night Fever: Club writing in* The Face *1980–1997*, London: Boxtree.

Bertoia, C. and Drakich, J. (1995) 'The Fathers' Rights Movement: contradictions in rhetoric and practice', in Marsiglio, W. (ed.), *Fatherhood: Contemporary Theory, Research, and Social Policy*, London: Sage.

Birch, D., White, M. and Kamali, F. (1999) 'Factors influencing alcohol and illicit drug use amongst medical students', University of Newcastle.

Bottoms, A. and Wiles, P. (1995) 'Crime and insecurity in the city', in Fijnaut, C., Goethals, J., Peters, T. and Walgrave, L. (eds), *Changes in Society, Crime and Criminal Justice in Europe*, 2 volumes, The Hague: Kluwer.

Bourdieu, P. (1984) *Distinction: A Social Critique of the Judgement of Taste*, Cambridge: Harvard University Press.

Boys, A. J., Fountain, J., Griffiths, P., Marsden, J., Stillwell, G. and Strang, J. (2000) *Drugs Decisions: A Qualitative Study of Young People*, London: Health Education Authority.

Brain, K., Parker, H. and Bottomley, T. (1998) *Evolving Crack Cocaine Careers*, London: Home Office Publications Unit.

Brake, M. (1985, this edition 1995) *Comparative Youth Culture: The Sociology of Youth Cultures and Youth Subcultures in America, Britain and Canada*, London: Routledge.

Branigan, P. and Wellings, K. (1999) 'Acceptance of the harm reduction message in London clubs and Underground system' *Drugs Education, Prevention and Policy* 6(3):389–99.

Breeze, J., Aldridge, J. and Parker, H. (2001) 'Unpreventable? How young people make and remake drugs decisions', Chapter 4 in Parker et al., *UK Drugs Unlimited: New Research and Policy Lessons on Illicit Drug Use*, Basingstoke: Palgrave.

Bussman, J. (1998) *Once in a Lifetime: The Crazy Days of Acid House and Afterwards*, London: Virgin.

Cahill, M. (1994) *The New Social Policy*, Oxford: Blackwell.

Calafat, A. (1998) *Nightlife in Europe and Recreative Drug Use*, Palma de Majorca: SONAR 98 IREFREA/European Commission.

Campbell, B. (1993) *Goliath: Britain's Dangerous Places*, London: Methuen.

Carrigan, T., Connell, R.W. and Lee, J. (1985) 'Toward a new sociology of masculinity' *Theory and Society*, 14 (5):551–604.

Census (1991) *The 1991 Census*, Crown Copyright. ESRC Purchase.

Champion, S. (ed.) (1997) *Disco Biscuits*, London: Sceptre/Hodder and Stoughton.

Clarke, J. and Critcher, C. (1985) *The Devil Makes Work: Leisure in Capitalist Britain*, Basingstoke: Macmillan.

Clarke, J., Hall, S., Jefferson, T. and Roberts, B. (1976) 'Subcultures, cultures and class: a theoretical overview', in Hall, S. and Jefferson, T. (eds), *Resistance Through Rituals: Youth Subcultures in Post-war Britain*, London: HarperCollins.

Clarke, J. and Jefferson, T. (1976) 'Working class youth cultures', in Mungham, G. and Pearson, G. (eds), *Working Class Youth Culture*, London: Routledge and Kegan Paul.

Coffield, F. and Gofton, L. (1994) *Drugs and Young People*, London: Institute for Public Policy Research.

Cohen, P. (1981, this edition 1990) 'Policing the working-class city', in Fitzgerald, M., McLennan, G. and Pawson, J., *Crime and Society: Readings in History and Theory*, London: Routledge.

Cohen, S. (ed.) (1971) *Images of Deviance*, Harmondsworth: Penguin.

Cohen, S. (1972, this edition 1973) *Folk Devils and Moral Panics: The Creation of the Mods and Rockers*, St Albans: Paladin.

Collin, M. and Godfrey, J. (1997) *Altered State: The Story of Ecstasy Culture and Acid House*, London: Serpent's Tail.

Collison, M. (1996) 'In search of the high life: drugs, crime, masculinity and consumption', *British Journal of Criminology*, 36 (3):428–44.

Connell, R.W. (ed.) (1993) *Theory and Society*, Special Issue on Masculinities, 22 (5).

Corkery, J. (2000a), *Drug Seizure and Offender Statistics, United Kingdom, 1998*, Home Office Statistical Bulletin 3/00, London: Research, Development and Statistics Directorate.

Corkery, J. (2000b) 'Snowed under – is it the real thing?' *Druglink* 15(3):12–16.

Crank, S., Dugdill, L., Peiser, B. and Guppy, A. (1999) 'Moving beyond the drugs and deviance issues: rave dancing as a health promoting alternative to conventional physical activity' conference paper at Club Health 2000, Royal Tropical Institute, Amsterdam.

Crome, I. (1999) 'Substance misuse and psychiatric co-morbidity: what are the issues?' *Drugs: Education, Prevention and Society* 6(2):151–75.

Curran, H. and Travill, R. (1997) 'Mood and cognitive effects of MDMA (ecstasy): weekend "high" followed by mid week low' *Addiction* 92(7):821–31.

Dorn, N. and South, N. (1990), 'Drug markets and law enforcement' *British Journal of Criminology, 30* (2):171–88.

Egginton, R., Aldridge, J. and Parker, H. (2001) 'Unconventional? Adolescent drug triers and users in England' Chapter 3 in Parker et al. *UK Drugs Unlimited: New Research and Policy Lessons on Illicit Drug Use*, Basingstoke: Palgrave.

Eisner, B. (1989) *Ecstasy: The MDMA Story*, Berkeley: Ronin.

EMCDDA (1999) *Extended Annual Report on the State of the Drugs Problem in the European Union*, Lisbon: European Monitoring Centre for Drugs and Drug Addiction.

ESPAD (1997) *Alcohol and Other Drug Use Among Students in 26 European Countries*, Swedish Council on Alcohol and Other Drugs, Stockholm.

Ettore, E. (1992) *Women and Substance Use*, Basingstoke: Macmillan.

Finch, J. (1999) 'Death dance of the disco' *Guardian* 23 January.

Fisher, M. (1994) 'Hello darkness, our new friend' *New Statesman and Society*, 11 March, 32–3.

Forsyth, A. (1998) 'A Quantitative Study of DanceDrug Use', PhD Glasgow University.

Foucault, M. (1961, this edition 1973) *Madness and Civilization: A History of Insanity in the Age of Reason*, New York: Vintage.

Foucault, M. (1984, this edition 1990) *The Care of the Self: The History of Sexuality Volume 3*, London: Penguin.

Fraser A., Gamble, L. and Kennett, P. (1992) 'Into the Pleasuredome ...', in Ashton, M. (ed.), *The Ecstasy Papers: A Collection of ISDD's Publications on the Dance Drugs Phenomenon*, London: ISDD.

Füredi, F. (1995) 'Is it a girl's world?', *Living Marxism*, May.

Furlong, A. and Cartmel, F. (1997) *Young People and Social Change*, Buckingham: Open University Press.

Garratt, S. (1998) *Adventures in Wonderland: A Decade of Club Culture*, London: Headline.

Garratt, S. and Baker, L. (1989) 'The We Generation: clubland's new era', *The Face*, December, reproduced in Benson, R. (ed.), (1997) *Night Fever: Club writing in* The Face *1980–1997*, London: Boxtree.

Garratt, S. and Taggart, C. (1990) 'Fighting for the right to party: HM Government versus Acid House, *The Face*, February', reproduced in Benson, R. (ed.), (1997) *Night Fever: Club Writing in* The Face *1980–1997*, London: Boxtree.

Generator, (1995) 2 (8), September, 'Who's who in jungle', 26–48.

Gibbins, J. and Reimer, B. (1999) *The Politics of Postmodernity: An Introduction to Contemporary Politics and Culture*, London: Sage.

Gilman, M. (1994), 'Football and drugs: two cultures clash' *International Journal of Drug Policy, 5* (1):40–8.

Gofton, L. (1990) 'On the town: drink and the "new lawlessness"' *Youth and Society, 29*, April, 33–9.

Gouzoulis-Mayfrank, E., Daumann, J., Tuchtenhagen, F., Pelz, S., Becker, S., Kunert, H., Fimm, B. and Sass, H. (2000) 'Impaired cognitive performance in drug free users of recreational ecstasy (MDMA)' *Journal of Neurological and Neurosurgical Psychiatry* 68:719–25.

Graham, J. and Bowling, B. (1995) *Young People and Crime* Home Office Research Study 145, London: Home Office.

Gray, R. and Thomas, B. (1996) 'Effects of cannabis abuse on people with serious mental health problems' *British Journal of Nursing* 5(4):230–3.

Greer, G. and Tolbert, R. (1986) 'Subjective reports of the effects of MDMA in a clincial setting' *Journal of Psychoactive Drugs* 18:319–27.

Griffiths, P., Vingoe, L., Jansen, K., Sherval, J., Lewis, R. and Hartnoll, R. (1997) *New Trends in Synthetic Drugs in the European Union*, Lisbon: EMCDDA.

Hall, S. and Jefferson, T. (eds), (1976), *Resistance Through Rituals: Youth Subcultures in Post-war Britain*, London: HarperCollins.

Hammersley, R., Ditton, J., Smith, I. and Short, E. (1999) 'Patterns of Ecstasy use by drug users' *British Journal of Criminology* 39(4):625–47.

Handy, C., Pater, R. and Barrowcliff, A. (1998) 'Drug use in South Wales: who uses Ecstasy anyway?' *Journal of Substance Misuse* 3:82–8.

Hanmer, J., Radford, J. and Stanko, E. (eds), (1989) *Women, Policing, and Male Violence: International Perspectives*, London: Routledge.

Hanna, J. (1988) *Dance, Sex and Gender: Signs of Identity, Dominance, Defiance and Desire*, Chicago: University of Chicago Press.

Hanna, K. (1999) 'On not playing dead', in Kelly, K. and McDonnell, E. (eds), *Stars Don't Stand Still in the Sky: Music and Myth*, London: Routledge.

Harrison, B. (1971) *Drink and the Victorians*, London: Faber and Faber.

Harrison, M. (1998) *High Society: The Real Voices of Club Culture*, London: Paitkus.

Hart, L. and Hunt, N.(1997) *Choosers Not Losers?*, Kent: Invecta Community Care NHS.

Haslam, D. (1999) *Manchester England: The Story of a Pop Cult City*, London: Fourth Estate.

HEA (1999) *Drug Use in England*, London: Health Education Authority.

Headon, J. (1994) 'Is jungle too ruff? Is jungle too moody, ruffneck and dangerous or is it the most popular, underground and "real" form of rave?' *Mixmag*, March, 36–7.

Health and Safety Executive (1998) *Drug Misuse at Work*, London: Health and Safety Executive.

Hebdige, D. (1976a) 'The meaning of mod', in Hall, S. and Jefferson, T., *Resistance Through Rituals: Youth Subcultures in Post-war Britain*, London: HarperCollins.

Hebdige, D. (1976b) 'Reggae, rastas and rudies', in Hall, S. and Jefferson, T. (eds), *Resistance Through Rituals: Youth Subcultures in Post-war Britain*, London: HarperCollins.

Hebdige, D. (1979, this edition 1994) *Subculture: The Meaning of Style*, London: Routledge.

Henderson, S. (1993a) 'Fun, fashion and frisson', *International Journal of Drug Policy*, 4 (3):122–9.

Henderson, (1993b) *Young Women, Sexuality and Recreational Drug Use: A Research and Development Project*, Final Report, Manchester: Lifeline.

Henderson, S. (1993c) 'Luvdup and de-elited: responses to drug use in the second decade', in Aggleton, P., Davies, P. and Hart, G. (eds), *AIDS: Facing the Second Decade*, London: Falmer.

Henderson, S. (1997) *Ecstasy: Case Unsolved*, London: Pandora.

Henderson, S. (1999) 'Drugs and culture: the question of gender', in South, N. (ed.), *Drugs: Cultures, Controls and Everyday Life*, London: Sage.

Henry, J. (1992) 'Ecstasy and the dance of death: Severe reactions are unpredictable' *British Medical Journal*, *305*, 4 July, 5–6.

Henry, J.A., Fallon, J.K., Kicman, A.T., Hutt, A.J., Cowan, D.A. and Forsling, M. (1998) 'Low-dose MDMA ("ecstasy") induces vasopressin secretion' *Lancet*, *351*, 13 June, 1784.

Hey, V. (1986) *Patriarchy and Pub Culture*, London: Tavistock.

Hills, G. (1993) 'Wonderland UK: why people take drugs and go to clubs', *The Face*, January, reproduced in Benson, R. (ed.), (1997), *Night Fever: Club writing in* The Face *1980–1997*, London: Boxtree.

Hindle, P. (1994) 'Gay communities and gay space in the city', in Whittle, S. (ed.), *The Margins of the City: Gay Men's Urban Lives*, Aldershot: Ashgate.

Hirst, J. and McCameley-Finney, A. (1994) *The Place and Meaning of Drugs in the Lives of Young People*, Sheffield: Sheffield Hallam University.

Hunt, G. and Satterlee, S. (1987) 'Darts, drink and the pub: the culture of female drinking' *Sociological Review*, *35* (3):575–601.

Huq, R. (1996) 'Asian kool? Bhangra and beyond', in Sharma, S., Hutnyk, J. and Sharma, A. (eds), *Dis-orienting Rhythms: The Politics of the New Asian Dance Music*, London: Zed.

Independent Inquiry (2000) *Drugs and the Law*, Report to the Independent Inquiry into the Misuse of Drugs Act 1971, Police Foundation, London.

Jackson, P. (1989) *Maps of Meaning: An Introduction to Cultural Geography*, London: Unwin Hyman.

James, M. (1997) *State of Bass – Jungle: The Story so Far*, London: Boxtree.

Johnson, B. (2000) Personal communication with leading authority on urinalysis and self reported drug taking in USA.

Jones, P.R.M., Hunt, M.J., Brown, T.P. and Norgan, N.G. (1986) 'Waist–hip circumference ratio and its relationship to age and overweight in British men' *Human Nutrition Clinical Nutrition* 40C: 239–47.

Jones, S. (1988) *Black Culture, White Youth: The Reggae Tradition from JA to UK*, London: Macmillan.

Journal of Chemical Dependency Treatment, (1992) Special edition, Lesbians and Gay Men: Chemical Dependency Treatment Issues.

Journal of Homosexuality, (1982) Special edition, Alcoholism and Homosexuality.

Klee, H. (1998) 'The Love of Speed: An analysis of the enduring attraction of amphetamine sulphate for British youth', in Power, R. (ed.) *Journal of Drug Issues*, Special Edition, Contemporary Issues Concerning Illicit Drug Use in the British Isles, *28* (1):33–55.

Klee, H. and Morris, J. (1994) 'Factors that lead young amphetamine misusers to seek help: implications for drug prevention and harm reduction' *Drugs: Education, Prevention and Policy* 1,(3):289–97.

Knight, I. (1984) *The Heights and Weights of Adults in Great Britain*. OPCS Social Survey Division, London: HMSO.

Kohn, M. (1992) *Dope Girls: The Birth of the British Drug Underground*, London: Lawrence and Wishart.

Kohn, M. (1997) 'The chemical generation and its ancestors: dance crazes and drug panics across eight decades' *International Journal of Drug Policy*, *8* (3):137–42.

Lenton, S., Boys, A. and Norcross, K. (1997) 'Raves, drugs and experience: drug use by a sample of people who attend raves in Western Australia' *Addiction* 92(10):1327–37.

Lewis, L. (1994) 'The inner Sydney gay dance party culture in the context of the HIV/AIDS pandemic: A qualitative analysis', unpublished PhD thesis, University of New South Wales.

Lewis, L. and Ross, M. (1995) *A Select Body: The Gay Dance Party subculture and the HIV/AIDS Pandemic*, London: Cassell.

Luke, C., Dewar, C., McGreevy, D. and Morris, H. (1999) 'A little night club medicine: the healthcare implications of clubbing' conference paper at Club Health 2000, Royal Tropical Institute, Amsterdam.

Lynsky, D. (1998) 'Ecstasy' *Mixmag*, June 1998.

McDermott, P. (1993), MDMA use in the north west of England, *International Journal of Drug Policy*, *4* (4):210–21.

McElrath, K. and McEvoy, K. (1999) *Ecstasy Use in Northern Ireland*, Belfast: Queen's University.

McGee, R., Williams, S., Poulton, R. and Moffitt, T. (2000) 'A longitudinal study of cannabis use and mental health from adolescence to early adulthood' *Addiction* 95(4):491–503.

McKeganey, N. and Norrie, J. (1999) 'Pre-teen drug users in Scotland' *Addiction Research* 7(6):493–507.

McKenna, T. (1992) *Food of the Gods: The Search for the Original Tree of Knowledge. A Radical History of Planets, Drugs and Human Evolution*, New York: Bantam.

McRobbie, A. (1999) 'Thinking with music', in Kelly, K. and McDonnell, E. (eds), *Stars Don't Stand Still in the Sky: Music and Myth*, London: Routledge.

Maher, L. (1997) *Sexed Work: Gender, Race, and Resistance in a Brooklyn Drug Market*, Oxford: Clarendon.

Makhoul, M., Yates, F. and Wolfson, S., (1998) 'A survey of substance use at a UK university: prevalence of use and views of students', *Journal of Substance Misuse* 3, pp. 119–24.

MAPS (1995) 'MDMA: A catalyst for healing my fears and depression' *Newsletter of the Multidisciplinary Association for Psychedelic Studies (MAPS)* 6(1) Autumn 1995. [WWW] http://www.maps.org/news-letters/v06n1/06114per.html

Marcus, T. (1994) Summer of jungle, in *Mixmag*, 2 (38) July, 33–6.

Marsh, P. and Fox Kibby, K. (1992) *Drinking and Public Disorder: A Report of Research Conducted for The Portman Group by MCM Research*, London: The Portman Group.

Marsiglio, W. (ed.) (1995) *Fatherhood: Contemporary Theory, Research, and Social Policy*, London: Sage.

Massey, D. (1994) *Space, Place and Gender*, Cambridge: Polity.

Maxwell, D.L., Polkey, M.I. and Henry, J.A. (1993) 'Hyponatraemia and catatonic stupor after taking "ecstasy"', *British Medical Journal, 307*, 27 November, 1399.

Mayhew, P. (1981, this edition 1990) 'On the number of costermongers and other street folk', in Fitzgerald, M., McLennan, G. and Pawson, J., *Crime and Society: Readings in History and Theory*, London: Routledge.

Measham, F. (1988) 'Men buy the beer and the leer: a case study of women and bar work', unpublished MA thesis, University of Warwick.

Measham, F. (2000) 'Locating leisure: feminist, historical and socio-cultural perspectives on young people's leisure, substance use and social divisions in 1990s British pubs and clubs', unpublished PhD thesis, University of Manchester.

Measham, F., Parker, H. and Aldridge, J. (1998a) 'The teenage transition: from adolescent recreational drug use to the young adult dance culture in Britain in the mid-1990s', in Power, R. (ed.), *Journal of Drug Issues*, Special Edition, Contemporary Issues Concerning Illicit Drug Use in the British Isles, *28* (1):9–32.

Measham, F., Parker, H. and Aldridge, J. (1998b) *Starting, Switching, Slowing, Stopping*, London: Home Office, Drugs Prevention Initiative, Green Series Paper 21.

Meikle, A., McCallum, C., Marshall, A. and Coster, G. (1996) *Drugs Survey on a Selection of Secondary School Pupils in the Glasgow Area Aged 13–16*, Glasgow: Glasgow Drugs Prevention Team.

Meltzer, H., Baljit, G., Petticrew, M. and Hinds, K. (1995) *OPCS Surveys of Psychiatric Morbidity in Great Britain*, London: HMSO.

Miles, S. (2000) *Youth Lifestyles in a Changing World*, Buckingham: Open University Press.

Mirrlees-Black, C., Budd, T., Partridge, S. and Mayhew, P. (1998) *The 1998 British Crime Survey: England and Wales*, Home Office Statistical Bulletin Issue 21/98, London: Research, Development and Statistics Directorate.

Mixmag (1998) 'Drug myths: is there any truth in those chemical tall tales?' *Mixmag*, September 1998.

Mixmag (1998) 'Ecstasy causes "permanent brain damage"' *Mixmag*, December 1998.

Moore, D. (1994) *The Lads in Action: Social Process in an Urban Youth Subculture*, Aldershot: Ashgate.

Moran, L. (2000) 'Homophobic violence: the hidden injuries of class', in Munt, S. (ed.), *Cultural Studies and the Working Class: Subject to Change*, London: Cassell.

Morris, S. (1998) *Clubs, Drugs and Doormen*, Crime Detection and Prevention Series Paper No. 86, London: Police Research Group.

Mungham, G. (1976) 'Youth in pursuit of itself', in Mungham, G. and Pearson, G. (eds), *Working Class Youth Culture*, London: Routledge and Kegan Paul.

Mungham, G. and Pearson, G. (eds), (1976) *Working Class Youth Culture*, London: Routledge and Kegan Paul.

Murdock, G. and McCron, R. (1976) 'Consciousness of class and consciousness of generation', in Hall, S. and Jefferson, T. (eds), *Resistance Through Rituals: Youth Subcultures in Post-war Britain*, London: HarperCollins.

Muzik, (1996) April, no.11, Mouth Off, letters, 166–7.

Muzik, (1996) June, no.13, Mouth Off, letters, 184–5.

Naylor T. (1996) 'Superclubs or superduds?', in *Wax*, 1 (4) July, 16–19.

Newcombe, R. (1991) *Raving and Dance Drugs: House Music Clubs and Parties in North-west England*, Liverpool: Rave Research Bureau.

Newcombe, R. (1992a) 'A researcher reports from the rave', in Ashton, M. (ed.), *The Ecstasy Papers: A Collection of ISDD's Publications on the Dance Drugs Phenomenon*, London: ISDD.

Newcombe, R. (1992b) *The Use of Ecstasy and Dance Drugs at Rave Parties and Nightclubs: Some Problems and Solutions*, Liverpool: 3D.

Newcombe, R. (1994) *Safer Dancing: Guidelines for Good Practice at Dance Parties and Nightclubs*, Liverpool: 3D.

Newcombe, R. and Johnson, M. (1999) 'Psychonautics: a model and method for exploring the effects of psychedelic drugs', paper presented to Club Health 2000 conference, Amsterdam, November.

Newsome, R. (1996) 'Exploring the jungle', in *City Life*, *300*, March 6–21, 10–11.

NHSDA (1999) *Factsheet: 1998 National Household Survey on Drug Abuse*, Washington: Office of National Drug Control Policy.

Office for National Statistics (1998) *Living in Britain: Results from the 1996 General Household Survey*, London.

Office of National Drug Control Policy (1999) *Review of 1999 Monitoring the Future*, Washington: Executive Office of the President.

O'Hagan, C. (1999) 'British dance culture: sub-genres and associated drug use', conference paper at Club Health 2000, Amsterdam, November, based on unpublished MSc thesis, Liverpool John Moores University.

Osgerby, B. (1998) *Youth in Britain since 1945*, Oxford: Blackwell.

Parker, H., Aldridge, J. and Egginton, R. (2001) *UK Drugs Unlimited: New Research and Policy Lessons on Illicit Drug Use*, Basingstoke: Macmillan.

Parker, H., Aldridge, J. and Measham, F. (1998) *Illegal Leisure: The Normalization of Adolescent Recreational Drug Use*, London: Routledge.

Pearson, G. (1983, this edition 1991) *Hooligan: A History of Respectable Fears*, Basingstoke: Macmillan.

Pedersen, W. and Skrondal, A. (1999) 'Ecstasy and new patterns of drug use: a normal population study' *Addiction* 94(11):1695–706.

Peroutka, S.J. (1990) *Ecstasy: The Clinical, Pharmacological and Neurotoxicological Effects of the Drug MDMA*. London: Kluwer Academic Publishers.

Perri, 6., Jupp, B., Perry, H. and Laskey, K. (1997) *The Substance of Youth*, York: Joseph Rowntree Foundation.

Petridis, A. (1996) 'How much Ecstasy do the British really take?' *Mixmag* 2, 62, July, 98–100.

Phoenix, J. (1999) 'Prostitutes, ponces and poncing: making sense of violence', in Seymour, J. and Bagguley, P. (eds), *Relating Intimacies: Power and Resistance*, Basingstoke: Macmillan.

Pirie, M. and Worcester, R. (1999) *The Next Leaders?*, London: Adam Smith Institute.

Plant, M.L. (1997) *Women and Alcohol: Contemporary and Historical Perspectives*, London: Free Association Books.

Plant, S. (1999) *Writing on Drugs*, London: Faber and Faber.

Plant, M.A. and Plant, M.L. (1992) *Risk Takers: Alcohol, Drugs, Sex and Youth*, London: Tavistock/Routledge.

Plant, M. and Miller, P. (2000) 'Drug use has declined among teenagers in the United Kingdom' *British Medical Journal* 320: 1536 (3 June).

POST (1996) *Common Illegal Drugs and their Effects: Cannabis, Ecstasy, Amphetamines and LSD*, London: Parliamentary Office of Science and Technology.

Power, R. (1995) *Coping with Illicit Drug Use*, London: Tufnell Press.

Ramsay, M. and Partridge, S. (1999) *Drug Misuse Declared in 1998: Results from the British Crime Survey*, Home Office Research Study 197, London: Home Office.

Ramsay, M. and Spiller, J. (1997) 'Drug misuse declared in 1996': Latest results from the British Crime Survey Home Office Research Study 172, London: Home Office.

Redhead, S. (1990) *The End-of-the-Century Party: Youth and Pop Towards 2000*, Manchester: Manchester University Press.

Redhead, S. (ed.) (1993) *Rave Off: Politics and Deviance in Contemporary Youth Culture*, Aldershot: Avebury.

Release (1997) *Release Drugs and Dance Survey*, London: Release.

Reynolds, S. (1997) 'Rave culture: living dream or living death?', in Redhead, S., Wynne, D. and O'Connor, J. (eds), *The ClubCultures Reader: Readings in Popular Cultural Studies*, Oxford: Blackwell.

Reynolds, S. (1998) *Energy Flash: A Journey through Rave Music and Dance Culture*, London: Macmillan.

Reynolds, S. (1999) 'Ecstasy is a science: techno-romanticism', in Kelly, K. and McDonnell, E. (eds), *Stars Don't Stand Still in the Sky: Music and Myth*, London: Routledge.

Reynolds, S. and Press, J. (1995) *The Sex Revolts: Gender, Rebellion and Rock 'n' Roll*, London: Serpent's Tail.

Riddiough, C. (1980) 'Culture and politics', in Mitchell, P. (ed.), *Pink Triangles: Radical Perspectives on Gay Liberation*, Boston: Alyson.

Rietveld, H. (1993) 'Living the dream', in Redhead, S. (ed), *Rave Off: Politics and Deviance in Contemporary Youth Culture*, Aldershot: Avebury.

Rogers, B. (1988) *Men Only: An Investigation of Men's Organisations*, London: Pandora.

Rojek, C. (2000) *Leisure and Culture*, Basingstoke: Macmillan.

Rose, D. and O'Reilly, K. (1998) *The ESRC Review of Government Social Classifications*, London: Office for National Statistics.

Rossow, I., Pape, H. and Wichstrom, L. (1999) 'Young, wet and wild? Associations between alcohol intoxication and violent behaviour in adolescence' *Addiction* 94(7):1017–31.

Ruggiero, V. (1994) 'Organised crime and drug economies', *International Journal of Drug Policy*, 5 (2):106–14.

Rust, F. (1969) *Dance in Society*, London: Routledge and Kegan Paul.

Saunders, N. (1993) *E for Ecstasy*, London: Nicholas Saunders.

Saunders, N. (1995) *Ecstasy and the Dance Culture*, London: Nicholas Saunders.

Saunders, N. (1997) *Ecstasy Reconsidered*, London: Nicholas Saunders.

Sauvages, F.B. de (1772) Nosologie Méthodique, Vol. VII, Lyons, quoted in Foucault, M. (1961, this edition 1973), *Madness and Civilization: A History of Insanity in the Age of Reason*, New York: Vintage.

Schifano, F., DiFuria, L., Forza, G., Minicuci, N. and Bricolo, R. (1998) 'MDMA ("ecstasy") consumption in the context of polydrug abuse: A report on 150 patients' *Drug and Alcohol Dependence* 52:85–90.

Scott, S. and Morgan, D. (eds), (1993) *Body Matters: Essays on the Sociology of the Body*, London: Falmer.

Scottish Drugs Forum, (1996) *The Survivors' Guide to Drugs and Clubbing*, Glasgow: Scottish Drugs Forum.

Scottish Office (1997) *Drug Misuse in Scotland: Findings from the 1993 and 1996 Scottish Crime Surveys*, Edinburgh: The Scottish Office Central Research Unit.

Segal, L. (1990) *Slow Motion: Changing Masculinities, Changing Men*, London: Virago.

Shapiro, H. (1999) 'Dances with drugs: pop music, drugs and youth culture', in South, N. (ed.) *Drugs: Cultures, Controls and Everyday Life*, London: Sage.

Sharma, S., Hutnyk, J. and Sharma, A. (eds), (1996) *Dis-orienting Rhythms: The Politics of the New Asian Dance Music*, London: Zed.

Shepherd, J. (1990) 'Violent crime in Bristol: an Accident & Emergency Department perspective' *British Journal of Criminology*, 30:(3).

Sherlock, J. (1993) 'Dance and the culture of the body', in Scott, S. and Morgan, D., *Body Matters: Essays on the Sociology of the Body*, London: Falmer.

Shewan, D., Dalgarno, P. and Reith, G. (2000) 'Perceived risk and risk reduction among ecstasy users: the role of drug, set and setting' *International Journal of Drug Policy* 10 (2000):431–53.

Shiner, M. and Newburn, T. (1997) 'Definitely, maybe not? The normalisation of recreational drug use amongst young people' *Sociology* V31, 3:511–29.

Shulgin, A.T. and Shulgin, A. (1991) *PIHKAL: A Chemical Love Story*, Berkeley: Transform.

Skeggs, B. (2000) 'The appearance of class: challenges in gay space', in Munt, S. (ed.), *Cultural Studies and the Working Class: Subject to Change*, London: Cassell.

Smitherman, G. (1997) '"The chain remain the same": communicative practices in the hip hop nation', *Journal of Black Studies*, 28 (1):3–25.

Spradley, J. and Mann, B. (1975) *The Cocktail Waitress: Woman's Work in a Man's World*, New York: John Wiley.

Stanley, C. (1997) 'Not drowning but waving: urban narratives of dissent in the wild zone', in Redhead, S., Wynne, D. and O'Connor, J. (eds), *The ClubCultures Reader: Readings in Popular Cultural Studies*, Oxford: Blackwell.

Stedman Jones, G. (1971, this edition 1984) *Outcast London: A Study in the Relationship between Classes in Victorian Society*, Harmondsworth: Peregrine.

Stedman Jones, G. (1983) *Languages of Class: Studies in English Working Class History 1832–1982*, Cambridge: Cambridge University Press.

Stevens, J. (1987, this edition 1993) *Storming Heaven: LSD and the American Dream*, London: Flamingo.

Swanton, O. (1998) 'Gangchester', in *Mixmag*, No. 81, February, 68–76.

Taylor, A. (1993) *Women Drug Users: An Ethnography of a Female Injecting Community*, Oxford: Clarendon.

Thomas, H. (1993) 'Psychiatric symptoms in cannabis users' *British Journal of Psychiatry* 163:141–9.

Thornton, S. (1995) *Club Cultures: Music, Media and Subcultural Capital*, Cambridge: Polity.

Tomsen, S. (1997) 'A top night: social protest, masculinity and the culture of drinking violence', *British Journal of Criminology*, 37 (1):90–102.

True, (1996) 7, March, 'Jungle vanguard: the establishment', 44–53.

Truman, C. (forthcoming) 'Somewhere under the rainbow – in search of lesbian space', *Journal of Urban Labour and Leisure*.

Tseloni, A. (1995) 'The modelling of threat incidence: evidence from the British Crime Survey', in Dobash, R.E., Dobash, R.P. and Noaks, L. (eds), *Gender and Crime*, Cardiff: University of Wales.

Van de Wyngaart, G., Braan, R., de Bruin, D., Fris, M., Maalste, N. and Verbraeck, H. (1998) *Ecstasy in het uitgaanscircuit*, Addiction Research Institute, Utrecht University.

Verheyden, S. and Curran, V. (1999) 'Predisposing factors for negative outcomes associated with use of MDMA (Ecstasy)' conference paper at Club Health 2000, Royal Tropical Institute, Amsterdam.

Walby, S. (ed.), (1999) *New Agendas for Women*, London: Macmillan.

Weaver, T., Renton, A. Stimson, G. and Tyrer, P. (1999) 'Several mental illness and substance misuse' *British Medical Journal* 318:137–8.

Webb, E., Ashton, C., Kelly, D. and Kamali, F. (1996) 'Alcohol and drug use in UK university students' *Lancet* 348:922–5.

Welsh, I. (1993, this edition 1996) *Trainspotting*, London: Minerva.

Welsh, I. (1994, this edition 1995) *The Acid House*, London: Vintage.

Welsh, I. (1995, this edition 1996) *Marabou Stork Nightmares*, London: Vintage.

Welsh, I. (1996) *Ecstasy: Three Tales of Chemical Romance*, London: Jonathan Cape.

Westwood, S. (1984) *All Day, Every Day: Factory and Family in the Making of Women's Lives*, London: Pluto Press.

Whittle, S. (ed.), (1994) *The Margins of the City: Gay Men's Urban Lives*, Aldershot: Arena.

Williams, C. (ed.), (1993) *Doing 'Women's Work': Men in Nontraditional Occupations*, London: Sage.

Williamson, S., Gossop, M., Powis, B., Griffiths, P., Fountain, J. and Strang, J. (1997) 'Adverse effects of stimulant drugs in a community sample of drug users' *Drug and Alcohol Dependence* 44:87–94.

Winstock, A. (2000) 'Risky behaviour and harm reduction amongst 1151 clubbers'. Paper to 11th International Conference on the Reduction of Drug Related Harm, Jersey.

Wise, J. (1997) 'Alcohol not drugs causes most problems at night clubs' *British Medical Journal* 315:1179.

Wright, L. (1999) *Young People and Alcohol*, London: Health Education Authority.

Wright, M.A. (1998) 'The great British ecstasy revolution', in McKay, G. (ed.), *DiY Culture: Party and Protest in Nineties Britain*, London: Verso.

Young, L. and Jones, R. (1997) *Young People and Drugs*, Liverpool: SHADO.

Zinberg, N.E. (1984) *Drug, Set, and Setting: The Basis for Controlled Intoxicant Use*, New Haven: Yale University Press.

Index

Compiled by Sue Carlton